OXFORD MEDICAL PUBLICATIONS

A Guide for New Principals

OXFORD GENERAL PRACTICE SERIES

A Guide for New Principals

Oxford General Practice Series • 35

MIKE PRINGLE

*General Practitioner and Professor of General Practice,
Nottingham University Medical School*

JACKY HAYDEN

Regional Adviser in General Practice, North-western Region

and

ANDREW PROCTER

General Practitioner, Gainsborough, Lincoln

OXFORD   NEW YORK   TOKYO
OXFORD UNIVERSITY PRESS
1996

Oxford University Press, Walton Street, Oxford OX2 6DP

Oxford   New York
Athens   Auckland   Bangkok   Bombay
Calcutta   Cape Town   Dar es Salaam   Delhi
Florence   Hong Kong   Istanbul   Karachi
Kuala Lumpur   Madras   Madrid   Melbourne
Mexico City   Nairobi   Paris   Singapore
Taipei   Tokyo   Toronto
and associated companies in
Berlin   Ibadan

Oxford is a trade mark of Oxford University Press

Published in the United States
by Oxford University Press Inc., New York

© Mike Pringle, Jacky Hayden, and Andrew Procter, 1996

A catalogue record for this book is available from the British Library

Library of Congress Cataloging in Publication Data
(Data available)

ISBN 0 19 262536 5

Typeset by Technical Typesetting Ireland
Printed in Great Britain
by Bookcraft (Bath) Ltd
Midsomer Norton, Avon

Contents

Contents

Preface

Entering a general practice as a young principal is never easy. The patients are all unfamiliar and may be grieving for the partner who left; the practice organization may be radically different from the training practice; and expectations and responsibilities are greatly increased.

The clinical task is daunting. Registrars usually have a caseload that predominantly consists of acute and short-term follow-up cases; as a principal the patients are often with you for decades, looking to you to share in their lives as your grow old together. The breadth and complexity of clinical care in general practice is enormous and for many patients a definitive diagnosis is not possible—coping with that uncertainty is a real challenge.

Being a partner means sharing all the financial and organizational responsibilities of a practice. A medium size fundholding practice will have a financial turnover in excess of £3m and will have over 40 members of staff. Taking on responsibility—albeit shared—for such an organization is a formidable proposition, and is a task for which many new principals are unprepared.

And then there is an even greater challenge—the challenge of personal growth. For general practitioners must improve the care they deliver year by year, must acquire methods for expanding their knowledge and skills, must adopt a rigorous quality assurance programme, and must contribute to the future of their discipline.

In the face of such challenges it is small wonder that many doctors retreat into hospital medicine or from medicine altogether. However, this book has been written by three general practitioners who do not regret their career choice; who regard general practice as the heart land of the health service; and who are convinced that, with the right support, it is an excellent environment in which a young doctor can exploit his or her potential.

This book is intended to be a part of that support. It looks at how primary care came to be what it is today and what it represents as a discipline. It then looks at the major problems a young principal will face and offers a range of solutions. Finally, it offers a number of visions in a section entitled 'getting it right'; these chapters are focused on real advice for the real world of general practice.

To work in a cohesive partnership with a strong, caring team in an appreciative community of patients over a period of time is a pleasure and a privilege. We hope that you find this book some help in achieving that dream.

Nottingham   M. P.
Manchester   J. H.
Gainsborough   A. P.
April 1996

Acknowledgements

The authors wish to acknowledge the invaluable help offered by all the young principals who assisted in their thinking, especially those that contributed to the study carried out across the Oxford and North West regions. That study informed the broad contents of this book and gave valuable insight into the nature of the problems with which we should deal.

Part 1

The context

1 The historical background to primary care in the UK

INTRODUCTION

An understanding of history is important for an appreciation of the origins and current features of primary care. Although history may be bunk, in Henry Ford's phrase, if you are building a new system from scratch, we continue to work in a health system and clinical discipline which is pervaded by history. Of necessity this general historic review is selective, and it lays special emphasis on general practice. In particular, it concentrates on those historical developments that effect the present. This chapter takes the story of general practice in a series of threads through to the late 1980s, when the storms of change swept through the whole health service—these are the subject of the next chapter.

THE MAJOR POLITICAL FORCES

Before the nineteenth century, medicine was a caring profession—it had little else to offer. There were valid therapeutic strategies available such as digitalis, but these were few among a plethora of remedies derived from the herbalistic lore of traditional healers, with the adjunct of rituals and beliefs that are now largely discredited.[1]

The Medicine Act of 1858 categorized the profession into three component parts. The physicians were those few doctors who worked in major British cities, tending to the wealthy for a living and voluntarily treating the poor in charity hospitals. The surgeons were derived from the artisans who had evolved from barber surgery to be the only interventionist (if brutally so) branch of medicine. These two groups were united in their determination to exclude the apothecaries from usurping their pre-eminence but they recognized the need to include the apothecaries within the formal professional structure.[1,2]

The apothecaries were the embodiment of medicine for most people in the country, dispensing advice and herbal remedies. The Medicine Act formalized a deal which has persisted to this day—the physicians and surgeons retained secondary care, but the apothecaries and their successors, general practitioners, had the right of referral, which meant they retained primary care. It can, therefore, be said that the former kept the hospitals, while the latter kept the patients.

This argument, cast nearly a century and a half ago, means that today's patients require a referral letter before gaining access to secondary care; and it is the basis of any ill-feeling concerning hospital out-reach, direct advertising by consultants to patients, and open access private clinics. In the middle of the second half of the twentieth century this convention seemed to be bending under enormous strain, but it has received a recent strong endorsement—the essence of fundholding is that non-emergency medical services are purchased by general practitioners and this reinforces their role in the referral process.

In 1912, Lloyd George's National Health Insurance Scheme further codified the separation between primary and secondary care by covering all workers who earned less than £160 per year for the cost of their general practitioner care and medicines, in addition to unemployment and sickness benefit. All families wanting to take advantage of this had to register with a general practitioner. Many general practitioners offered a scheme whereby those not covered by the National Health Insurance Scheme could join a sick club and be covered for a few pence a week.[3] The system of patient registration persists, largely unaltered, to this day, and contributes one of the remarkable features of British general practice—the registered list means that there is a long-term relationship and responsibility between doctors and individual patients, and between practices and populations of patients.

The creation of the National Health Service in 1948[4] following the Beveridge Report[5] further increased the differentiation between secondary and primary care. Many hospitals were heavily dependent on charity and after the second world war were desperately short of funds. Many consultants continued in the eighteenth century model of seeing those who could afford their services in their private rooms, but dedicating much of their time, for small payment, to public hospitals.

Their NHS contracts were designed to reflect this state of affairs, by offering a salary for their NHS hospital work, but allowing time for them to pursue their private practice. It was this concession wrung from the Government which brought the consultants around to accepting the new service. They saw the possibility of continuing their tradition of private practice with their 'charity' work, on which their reputations were built, now adequately paid.

By contrast, most general practitioners had few wealthy patients and were heavily dependent on their work with the less well off. Their contract simply replaced the individual patient as the payee with the state. Since the state may be regarded as a more regular and reliable payer, it might be thought that general practitioners would welcome the National Health Service. This was not the case since many suspected that they would be low in the financial and hierarchial pecking order in the new system. Their worst fears were, of course, to be confirmed. The general practitioner contract in the early years of the National Health Service involved a capitation payment for each registered patient, with a fixed payment for practice expenses. This preserved the independent contractor status of general practitioners, but institutionalized some of the worst features of the pre-NHS days.[6]

In the 1950s, general practice declined.[7,8] This was also happening in many other European countries and in North America,[1] but in Britain it was not simply the result of a cultural shift towards a belief in technological medicine, nor due to patients by-passing their general practitioner. The right of referral kept the patients in primary care, where the workload was daunting.[7] The situation was wonderfully described by a visiting doctor from New Zealand, Joseph Collings, who was so dismayed by what he saw that he submitted a detailed description to the Lancet in 1950.[9]

The reason for the decline in primary care was two-fold. Firstly, the general practice contract acted as a disincentive to investment by the doctors—investment in premises or personnel only served to reduce their income. The second reason was that the state gave a higher priority to secondary care. General practitioners were poorly paid and ill-supported. Some suggested that any medical graduate worth his or her salt wished to enter the hospital service, and to enter general practice was to fall off the medical ladder.[9]

The 1966 General Practice Charter[10] was an inspired response to this decline. Kenneth Robinson, the Minister of Health, realized that the core of the health service—primary care—was rotten and that it required a new contract and new money. He set in train the renaissance of general practice, with increased investment in premises, staff, and equipment and a long-term rise in general practitioner earnings. He also, of course, contributed to the subsequent dramatic increase in the national expenditure on health.

The 1965 charter offered partial reimbursements of staff costs for a defined range of personnel. These included receptionists, dispensers, and nurses, but not practice managers, chiropodists, or physiotherapists. One can only wonder at what primary care might look like now if the list had differed. But the 70 per cent reimbursement was a major incentive in the staffing of primary care and the creation of primary health care teams.[11]

The rent reimbursement included in the charter was altered over the years to include, first, the payment of a notional rent for those practices that owned their own premises and then the Cost Rent Scheme for those developing new premises. These are embellishments on the basic philosophy of the charter—that primary care development was a partnership between the profession and Government, and that the latter had to bear its full financial burden.

Meanwhile, the hospitals reached their zenith in the 1970s. A major district hospital building programme coupled with the arrival of new, and expensive, technological investigations and treatments led to a dramatic increase in expenditure on secondary care. While it still lagged behind that of other major western countries, the accelerating expenditure led many to question the balance in medical care.[2] The coincident interest in complementary medicine[12] highlighted a dual yearning for both simple remedies and heart transplants.

The first central response was to re-organize the NHS in 1983[13] in an attempt to increase control over the health system and resource decisions. This was followed by the abolition of the Area Health Authorities in 1986,[14] a move designed to further increase direct control. The increase in expenditure on drugs and hospital care continued, however, unabated. By the late nineteen eighties, the Government had decided that it was getting the worst of both worlds—increasing expenditure and criticism when any under-provision was apparent. In the 1987 general election, the Conservative Government found itself, despite greatly increased funding in real terms of the health services, facing major political questions, especially concerning operations on children.

Following that election, the Government started a review process which was to leave no stone of the NHS untouched. If the situation immediately prior to the reforms is recalled, it was characterized by increasing waiting lists for operations; notable examples of 'shroud waving' by doctors and the press; and a serious loss of morale, especially in secondary care. The NHS reforms of the 1990s and more recent developments in general practice are described in the next chapter. The remainder of this chapter will examine four important trends which have a clear bearing on general practice today—the developments of an educational base; quality assurance; technology; and academic general practice.

VOCATIONAL TRAINING AND THE MRCGP

That general practice had become by the 1980s a relative political backwater was due largely to its success. From being the embarrassment of the 1950s health services, primary care had become its stable centre, around which the maelstrom of secondary care swirled. This transformation was not just due to developments such as the new charter, although that should not be underestimated.

The creation of the College of General Practitioners in 1951 (it did not achieve Royal status until 1967) was, in retrospect, a key turning point.[15] Long resisted by the other Royal Colleges, the formation of an academic organization to represent the aspirations of general practitioners offered a chimera that could motivate the activists in the profession. And it was not long before substance replaced the chimera.

The first substantial success for the Royal College of General Practitioners (RCGP) ideals came when the Todd Committee[16] examined medical education in the mid-1960s. The college's evidence argued for a common pre-registration year, and then four years of vocational training. This suggestion was remarkably radical for a time when doctors were free to enter general practice immediately after their pre-registration year; and higher professional training was the pre-serve of hospital specialities. The final Todd report plumped for a three year basic training for every doctor after registration, with specialist training continu-ing for two years afterwards. It was largely ignored in the other Royal Colleges but in general practice this recommendation was seized on as a means to establishing standards.

The RCGP was instrumental in setting up the early vocational training schemes and in establishing their success. In 1964, after several years of manouvering, the College established a Working Party on vocational training which culminated in 1967 with the publication of a report, *The implementation of vocational training*.[17] A prototype vocational training scheme was then inaugu-rated in Wessex, followed by schemes up and down the country.[18] It took until 1974 before the Conference of Local Medical Committees was able to support the concept of vocational training.

In the only legislation that proscribes any higher professional training for any branch of medicine, parliament approved in November 1976 a Bill which required the completion of training before entry into general practice as a principal. This law lays down that from 1981 every doctor entering general practice should have done a three year period of vocational training, and should have a certificate of satisfactory completion of vocational training.

By the time of the vocational training legislation, the national supervisory role had been transferred to the Joint Committee on Postgraduate Training for General Practice (JCPTGP). Although this body is housed in the RCGP headquarters in Princes Gate, London, and the College has equal representation with the General Medical Services Committee of the British Medical Association, the JCPTGP is not a College committee.[19] The local organization of vocational training passed to the Regional Advisers in General Practice who are university appointments. Although many of them have strong links to the College and support it in its endeavours, the making of vocational training mandatory by legislation prised it out of the RCGP's grasp.

However, the college already had another well established task. The early members of the RCGP joined by subscribing. Fellows were selected on the recommendation of colleagues. In 1965, the Council of the College decided that entry into the College should be by examination—and since 1968 it has been almost the only route to full membership. The MRCGP examination is the only College entrance examination which is validated and continually appraised.[20] It has developed methodologies that include multiple choice questions, a critical reading paper, and now a clinical component in which consultation skills are assessed. The College has now endorsed that 'trainees' should be called 'registrars'.

Two substantial cohorts of committed general practitioners thus created by the College—the trainers and examiners—were the power houses for the reformation of primary care. Whatever else the College has produced in its first forty years—and one must not ignore its journal and publications, its political manoeuvring, and its quality initiatives—its most remarkable success has been a cultural one. It proved to general practitioners themselves, the Government, other specialisms, and the public that general practitioners have the skills, knowledge, and commitment to be a real discipline within the medical profession.

QUALITY ASSURANCE

Another powerful thread in recent years has a long but weak history—quality assurance, often known in primary care as medical or clinical audit. The early days of hospital medicine were characterized by a search for information. In the absence of effective therapeutic interventions in the major diseases, the emphasis was on correct diagnosis and a premium was placed on the clinical examination of a patient. The diagnoses made clinically could, all too soon in many cases, be directly compared to abnormal structural findings after death. The collegiate nature of hospitals combined with a pursuit for diagnostic accuracy provided the first two examples of medical audit in action—the grand round and the post-mortem. Both are based on individual cases, are conducted in a spirit of peer review, and they served to increase knowledge as well as standards.

Such methods were, however, unsuited to primary care, where most patients did not have the florid physical signs seen in secondary care, where peer scrutiny was not present, and where most patients did not pass quickly into the hands of the undertakers. It must also be acknowledged that the patrician nature of the doctor–patient relationship served to stifle any consumer demands for quality. Consumerism was late to arrive on the British agenda.

This was not the case in North America where the sudden demand for medical care in the first decade of this century led to a dramatic drop in the standards of medical education.[21] Doctors were taken into medical schools without a secondary education and turned loose on the populace after two years of lectures—resulting in a 1910 demand for auditing of standards of care.[22] Subsequently, Americans have often shown the United Kingdom the lead in medical audit, especially in secondary care.[21] Their most significant export has been the thinking of Avadis Donebedian who postulated the now familiar triad of structure, process, and outcome.[23, 24] They continue to innovate in inter-hospital comparisons which have developed further than in Britain.

Meanwhile British hospitals developed their experience with perinatal mortality meetings into systematic reviews of hospital records[25] and the Confidential Enquiry into Perioperative Deaths (CEPOD).[26] The emphasis continued to be firmly in the tradition of case based audits centred around the examination of sample medical records.[27] In hospitals, it is possible to gather together substantial numbers of patients with particular diagnoses, many of which may be infrequent in the general population. Early medical research is filled with descriptions of such cohorts and these reports expanded the gaining of knowledge from the particular patient to the cohort. The application of medical audit to such groups is, however, still underdeveloped in secondary care.

It was inevitable that primary care would become involved in medical audit eventually. Early audits looked at workload, prescribing patterns, morbidity, patient satisfaction, referral, and consultation rates.[8, 28-34] From these it was immediately clear that medical auditing was taking a new course—to look at particular aspects of the care of substantial generic groups of patients rather than concentrating on individual cases. This was partly an opportunistic reaction to the availability of such groups of patients and their medical records, but it was also a defensive posture. To look at groups of patients and describe their care was seen as less threatening than case based audit which would involve judgements. As Curtis reported in 1974: 'There is no tradition of reviewing the general practitioner's work in Britain and there would be strong resistance to it'.[28]

In 1972 McWhinney, a Canadian, began to espouse medical audit as a facet of continuing education: 'As an educational experience a good system of medical audit is worth any number of postgraduate courses'.[35] This challenge was taken up by a number of enthusiasts[36, 37] who began to formulate a theoretical framework for primary care audit which might be seen as less personally threatening. The process was facilitated by the burgeoning of group practices[38] which involved their members in shared responsibility. The clinical record thus became more accessible to peers and much of the fear was eroded.

A major facilitator for quality assurance in primary care was the arrival of vocational training. As standards were introduced into the vocational training schemes, prospective trainers were required to audit their medical records system and to demonstrate their quality against nationally agreed standards.[18] The registrars (previously vocational trainees) were encouraged to undertake audits in the practices and national prizes were given for the best. Vocational training was clearly linked to the peer group status and financial rewards of being a vocational trainer and auditing was therefore accepted as a necessary inconvenience. It is widely accepted anecdotally that the standards of records required for accreditation for training had a dramatic and lasting effect on both the quality of those records and the manner in which they were viewed and used within the practices.

The belief of the enthusiasts that audit was a necessary part of quality of care was undermined by the lack of evidence that audit resulted in improvements in care. From the early 1970s scepticism was rife,[39-43] but the evidence has been mounting that involvement in audit—ownership of audit—does in fact improve care.[43,44] This argument has, however, been overtaken by events. Once medical audit entered the political sphere—medico-political and frankly political—considerations of efficacy became secondary. The prime issue became to demonstrate the care that general practice was delivering, as much from defensive posture as from one of quality of care.[45]

In 1983, the innovators of vocational training, embodied in the then Chairman of the Council of the Royal College of General Practitioners, Donald Irvine, developed the College's 'quality initiative'.[46] In primary care as a whole it was largely greeted with pious hopes and atavistic apathy. However, members of the College Council began to audit their practices and publish the results.[47,48]

The extraordinary foresight of the quality initiative is demonstrated by its two principal aims:

Within general practice as a whole each of us should be able to achieve the following broad aims within the next ten years:

1. To be able to say, at any moment in time, what the content of our work is and therefore what services each of us provides.

2. To incorporate standard setting and performance review as an integral and effective part of our professional lives.[49]

In 1985, the College published *What sort of doctor?*[50] This working party report set out a scheme for exchange practice visits in which both the visited and the visitor could look at the practice's performance and learn from it. As a first practical guide to peer review it was a radical concept which floundered for two reasons—it was culturally before its time, and it required substantial effort for little immediate, secular reward.

The 'what sort of doctor?' deliberations were not, however, wasted. The College built on them to develop the principles and finally, in 1989, the reality of Fellowship by Assessment.[51]

A series of essential criteria were developed, all based on patient care, that were both objective and auditable. An applicant knows in advance the standard to be met and all criteria must be met.

The concurrent tightening up throughout the 1980s of vocational training practice visits and assessments has helped to create a culture of critical evaluation in many practices in Britain. This has been led by the College and the General Medical Services Committee through the Joint Committee on Post-Graduate Training for General Practice. In 1992, the General Medical Services Committee published the results of its comprehensive survey of general practitioner attitudes,[52] and found that only 33 per cent of respondents disagreed with the statement that 'an accreditation system in general practice is long overdue'.

General practice has not, of course, been operating in the quality field in a vacuum—hospital colleagues have been doing high quality audits.[26,27,53] But it is true to say that primary care has shown the most significant cultural shift.[54] Many practices have been examining their care and compiling practice reports[55] which focused on quality; and in the late 1980s these had become commonplace.

INFORMATION TECHNOLOGY—THE NEW FORCE

This historical thread is altogether more recent, but it is an important component of the general practice we all currently inhabit. Among the many vaunted revolutions in medicine of the past decade, the undramatic but relentless advent of computerization in general practice has been one of the most profound and radical. In the 1991 Department of Health survey of computer use, 63 per cent of practices had a computer with a prediction of at least 86 per cent by 1995.[56]

Computers did not of course arrive into a vacuum. In the 1960s age–sex registers[57] were followed by disease registers.[58-61] By 1985, a survey in the West Midlands found that 52 per cent of practices had registers which they used for screening and surveillance, disease recording, and research.[62] As early as 1963 the problems of diagnostic labels in general practice were acknowledged[60] and this led to the development of the RCGP classification of disease.[63,64] The importance of these two synergistic developments cannot be underestimated. Without the instillation of a culture that accepted the need and utility of sub-population identification, and the tool with which to code illness, the introduction of computers would have been long delayed.

It is difficult to pin-point the first use of computers in general practice, but the honour must probably go to Abrams who described a functioning system in 1968.[65,66] Grene was achieving computer recalls in 1971.[67] It was not until the Exeter Community Health Services Computer Project that a system functionally recognizable as a practice computer system of today was developed and computers reached the general practice consciousness.[68,69] Almost simultaneously a similar system, based on a mainframe with land lines to the practices, was developed in Oxford under the charismatic directorship of Perry.[70,71]

By the late 1970s micro-computers were being introduced and the prospect of widespread, if ruinously expensive, computer use began to be discussed. The report of a working party of the Royal College of General Practitioners, *Computers in primary care*, was published in 1980[72] which set out one particularly far-sighted idea: 'The development of general practice computer systems and the parallel development of clinical standards to which the whole profession is already committed are closely inter-related'.

When the Department of Trade and Industry announced the 'Micros for general practitioners scheme' in 1982 there were about 50 practices using computers. The 140 systems which were to be installed represented, therefore, a quantum leap forward. That 1015 practices applied for places on the scheme illustrated the increasing interest in computing among general practitioners.[73,74]

With the arrival of the 'No cost option' computer systems in 1987,[75] primary care computing had another external shot in the arm. Two companies, VAMP and Meditel, offered general practices minimal cost computer systems of a high specification if they would allow their data to be aggregated centrally for research (which to all intents and purposes meant post-marketing surveillance of drugs).

The effect of the 'No cost option' was dramatic. While only 10 per cent of practices were computerized in 1987,[76] this was to take off dramatically over the next three years—19 per cent in 1988, 28 per cent in 1989, and 47 per cent in 1990.[56] The benefits were not just in the penetration of computerization but also in the range and intensity of data recording.

Practices received regular feedback on data quality and partners were encouraged to at least comply with the minimum standards of the two suppliers.

Following a report from the Joint Computing Group in 1988,[77] the Department of Health negotiated the purchase by the Crown of the copyright to the Read Codes.[78] A direct consequence was the creation of the National Health Service Centre for Coding and Classification in Loughborough with James Read as its first director. The Read Codes are the only ones which allow for a full coding of the clinical consultation and they open the vista of the electronic medical record.[79] By the time of the NHS reforms in the late 1980s, the electronic building blocks were in place to allow for the other great medical revolution of the last decade of the twentieth century—information handling.

ACADEMIC GENERAL PRACTICE

'Evidence based medicine' is now a vogue concept. While doctors have always striven to offer medicine based on scientific findings, the behavior of clinicians has always been founded on a combination of science-based knowledge, misinterpreted and inaccurate research results, traditional beliefs and personal beliefs, with the latter two often resulting from following the example of those we respect. In general practice the knowledge base, such as it is, is often borrowed from other disciplines; many areas of our practice have yet to be explored fully.

In a recent paper, Sweeney and colleagues showed that the evidence for the use of warfarin in atrial fibrillation was derived from small, heavily selected groups of patients researched in secondary care.[80] They question, rightly, the extent to which such findings are applicable to the population of patients with atrial fibrillation that we encounter in primary care. This paper illustrates the need for all disciplines to define their own skills and knowledge, to prepare its own members, and to undertake its own research.

At first, the research base for general practice was generated by individuals who happened to be general practitioners. We lay claim to Jenner and his work on a vaccine for smallpox and to Mackenzie who undertook seminal research in cardiology. Pickles showed the potential for epidemiology by studying infectious diseases in the Yorkshire dales, and was the first researcher of note to be recognizable as a general practitioner of today. When the Royal College of General Practitioners was formed in 1952 there were others carrying on the tradition—Pinsent, Fry, Hodgkin—but there was no research culture to speak of.

While many medical students were exposed to general practice, usually for a few days, it was not until 1956 that the first university department of general practice was established—in Edinburgh—and 1963 before the first professor of general practice was appointed—again in Edinburgh. The first chair in England was created at Manchester in 1972 and by 1995 all British medical schools bar two—Oxford and Cambridge—have a professor of general practice.

While we can claim a quarter of century as a credible academic discipline, the physicians (College of Physicians since 1518) and surgeons (College of Surgeons since 1810) have a considerable march on us. Further, the funding for academic general practice has never been very secure and curriculum time has had to be fought for.[81, 82] Despite this, the British Journal of General Practice (formerly the Journal of the Royal College of General Practitioners) is the primary care journal with the greatest citation rate in the world and the proportion of research funds entering our discipline is burgeoning.

As the GMC's document *Tomorrow's doctors*[83] puts increasing emphasis on community based teaching and the new SIFT proposals[84] plan to move resources into primary care teaching, we find ourselves with a young but vital discipline which is ready to take its place alongside the traditional hospital based disciplines. We do have, however, a formidable task still to address if we are to teach medicine to medical students in primary care; if we are to re-introduce inter-personal and holistic care at the centre of the curricula; and if we are to define the knowledge base for our discipline.

CONCLUSIONS

This chapter has looked at some of the predominant strands in the historical development of primary care. The wider political field has been characterized by the near extinction of general practice followed by its reformation. This resurgence was supported by the creation of the college, the MRCGP examination, and vocational training. Three other historical threads have come to dominate the current landscape of general practice. The first, quality assurance, has a long tradition but acceptance into the mainstream culture was more recent; and the second, general practice computing, is a relative newcomer which will be increasingly influencing day to day practice in the next decade. Finally, the recent emergence of general practice as an academic discipline offers us a future as a credible discipline in the health service.

REFERENCES

1. Tudor Hart, J. *A new kind of doctor*. London: Merlin Press, 1988.
2. Marinker, M. *Developments in primary health care*. In: A new NHS act for 1996? London: Office of Health Economics, 1984.
3. *Trends in general practice*. Ed: Fry, J. London: Royal College of General Practitioners, 1977.
4. Minister of Health and Minister of Health for Scotland. *A National Health Service*. London: HMSO, 1944.
5. *Social insurance and allied services report* (*Beveridge Report*). London: HMSO, 1942.
6. Pater, J. E. *The making of the National Health Service*. London: King Edward's Hospital Fund for London, 1981.
7. Hadfield, S. J. A field survey of general practice. *British Medical Journal*, 1953; **2**: 683–706.
8. Pinsent, R. J. F. H. The future of general practice. *Lancet*, 1950; **1**: 917–18.
9. Collings, J. S. General practice in England today, a reconnaissance. *Lancet*, 1950; **1**: 555–85.
10. British Medical Association. A new contract for general practitioners; a charter for the family doctor service. *British Medical Journal*, 1965; **2**: 889–891.
11. Hasler, J. Partners in practice: the primary health care team: history and contractual farces. *British Medical Journal*, 1992; **305**: 232–4.
12. Petroni, P. Partners in practice: beyond the boundaries: relationship between general practice and complementary medicine. *British Medical Journal*, 1992; **305**: 564–6.
13. Department of Health and Social Security. *Patients first: consultative paper on the structure and management of the NHS in England and Wales*. London: HMSO, 1979.
14. Griffiths, B. *The NHS Management inquiry report*. London: DHSS 1983.
15. Gray, D. P. History of the Royal College of General Practitioners—the first 40 years. *British Journal of General Practice*, 1992; **42**: 29–35.
16. *The report of the Royal Commission on medical education* (*Todd report*). London: HMSO, 1968.
17. *The implementation of vocational training*. London: Royal College of General Practitioners, 1967.
18. Irvine, I. *Teaching practices—report from general practice 15*. London: Royal College of General Practitioners, 1972.
19. Hasler, J. History of vocational training for general practice: the 1970s and 1980s. *Journal of the Royal College of General Practitioners*, 1989; **39**: 338–41.
20. Walker, H. J. Quantity, quality and controversy. *Journal of the Royal College of General Practitioners*, 1983; **33**: 545–6.

21. Lembcke, P.A. Evaluation of medical audit. *JAMA*, 1967, **199**: 543–500.
22. Flexner, A. *Medical education in United States and Canada—report to the Carnegie Foundation*. New York: Merrymount Press, 1910.
23. Donabedian, A. The methods and findings of quality assessment and monitoring—an illustrative analysis. In *Explorations in quality assurance and medical malpractice*. Michigan: Health Administration Press, 1985.
24. Donabedian, A. Evaluating the quality of medical care. *Millbank Memorial Fund Quarterly*, 1966; **44**: 166–204.
25. Heath, D. A. Random review of hospital patients' records. *British Medical Journal*, 1990; **300**: 651–2.
26. Buck, N., Devlin, H. B., and Lunn, J. N. *The report of a confidential enquiry into perioperative deaths*. London: Nuffield Provincial Hospitals Trust and Kind Edward's Hospital Fund for London, 1987.
27. Hopkins, A. Approaches to medical audit. *J. Epid. Comm. Health*, 1991; **45**: 1–3.
28. Curtis, P. Medical audit in general practice. *Journal of the Royal College of General Practitioners*, 1974; **24**: 607–611.
29. Forsyth, G. and Logan, R. L. F. Studies in medical care. In *Towards a measure of medical care*. Oxford: Oxford University Press, 1962.
30. Carwright, A. *Patients and their doctors—a study in general practice*. London: Routledge & Kegan Paul, 1967.
31. Seiler, E. R. Immunisation in general practice—analysis of some of the factors involved. *Journal of the Royal College of General Practitioners*, 1967; **13**: 197–204.
32. Korsch, B. B., Gozzi, E. K., and Francis, V. Gaps in doctor-patient communication. 1. Doctor-patient interaction and satisfaction. Paediatrics; 42: 855–871.
33. Drury, M. and Kuenssberg, E. V. Inquiry into administrative activities in general practice. *British Medical Journal*. 1970; **4**: 42–4.
34. Honnogsbaus, F. Quality in general practice—a commentary on the quality of care provided by general practitioners. *Journal of the Royal College of General Practitioners*, 1972; **22**: 429–51.
35. McWhinney, I. R. Medical audit in North America. *British Medical Journal*, 1972; **2**: 277–9.
36. Capstick, L. Need for pilot studies in general practice. *British Medical Journal*, 1974; **1**: 278–80.
37. Mourin, K. Audit in general practice. *Journal of the Royal College of General Practitioners*, 1975; **25**: 682–3.
38. Central Health Services Council. *The organisation of group practice*. London: HMSO, 1971.
39. Fessel, W. J. and Van Brunt, E. E. Assessing quality of care from the medical record. *New England Journal of Medicine*, 1972; **296**: 134–8.
40. Marson, W. S., Morrell, D. C., Watkins, C. J., and Zander, I. Measuring the quality of general practice. *Journal of the Royal College of General Practitioners*, 1973; **23**: 23–31.
41. Brook, R. H. and Appel, F. A. Quality of care assessment: choosing a method. *New England Journal of Medicine*, 1973; **288**: 1323–9.
42. Putnam, R. W. and Curry, L. Impact of patient care appraisal on physician behavior in the office setting. *Can. Med. Assoc. J.*, 1985; **132**: 1025–9.
43. Anderson, C. M., Chambers, S., Clamp, M., Dunn, I. A., McGhee, M. G., Sumner, K. R., and Wood, A. M. Can audit improve patient care? Effects of studying digoxin in general practice. *British Medical Journal*, 1988; **297**: 113–14.
44. Horder, J., Bosenquet, N., and Stocking, B. Ways of influencing the behaviour of general practitioners. *Journal of the Royal College of General Practitioners*, 1986, **36**: 517–21.

45. Walters, W. H. R., Kelt, J., and Lunn, J. E. Attitudes to audit. *Journal of the Royal College of General Practitioners*, 1983; **33**: 263–6.

46. Irvine, D. Quality of care in general practice. *Journal of the Royal College of General Practitioners*, 1983; **33**: 521–3.

47. Anonymous. *Quality of care initiatives by members of the Council*. London: Royal College of General Practitioners, 1984.

48. Anonymous. *Quality of care initiatives by members of the Council*. London: Royal College of General Practitioners, 1986.

49. Royal College of General Practitioners. *Quality in general practice—policy statement 2*. London: Royal College of General Practitioners, 1985.

50. What sort of doctor working party. *What sort of doctor?* London: Royal College of General Practitioners, 1985.

51. Royal College of General Practitioners. *Fellowship by assessment—occasional paper 50*. London: Royal College of General Practitioners, 1990.

52. Electoral reform society. *Your choices for the future—a survey of general practitioner opinion*. London: General Medical Services Committee of the British Medical Association, 1992.

53. Royal College of Physicians of London. *Medical audit—a first report*. London: Royal College of Physicians, 1989.

54. Marinker, M. (ed.) *Medical audit and general practice*. London: British Medical Journal, 1990.

55. Pringle, M. Practice reports. In *Medical audit and general practice* (ed., Marinker, M.) London: British Medical Journal, 1990.

56. Department of Health. *GP Computing, 1991 survey*. NHS Management Executive, London, 1991.

57. Pinsent, R. J. F. H. The evolving age–sex register. *Journal of the Royal College of General Practitioners*, 1968; **16**: 127–34.

58. Burdon, J. F. Display by spectrum. *Journal of the Royal College of General Practitioners*, 1961; **4**: 106.

59. Eimerl, T. S. Organised curiosity. *Journal of the Royal College of General Practitioners*, 1960; **3**: 246–52.

60. Watford, P. A. The practice index. *Journal of the Royal College of General Practitioners*, 1963; **6**: 225–32.

61. Morgan, R. H. The use of an age–sex register as a practice index. *Journal of the Royal College of General Practitioners*, 1965; **9**: 64.

62. Cooper, R. F. Do most practices have an age–sex register? Results of the West Midlands age–sex register study. *British Medical Journal*, 1985; **291**: 1391–3.

63. Royal College of General Practitioners. Classification of disease. *Journal of the Royal College of General Practitioners*, 1963; **6**: 219–24.

64. Royal College of General Practitioners. *Classification of diseases, problems and procedures 1984*. Occasional Paper 26. RCGP, London: 1984.

65. Abrams, M. E. A computer general practice and health information system. *Journal of the Royal College of General Practitioners*, 1968; **16**: 415–27.

66. Abrams, M. E. Computer terminals in a health centre. *Health Trends*, 1972; **4**: 18–20.

67. Grene, J. D. Automated recall in general practice. *Journal of the Royal College of General Practitioners*, 1971; **21**: 352–5.

68. Bolden, K. J. Computers in the consulting room. *Update*, 1981: 1627–33.

69. Bradshaw-Smith, J. H. The role of the computer in general practice. *The Practitioner*, 1982; **226**: 1211–3.

70. Perry, J. Medical information systems in general practice—a community health project. *Proceedings of the Royal Society of Medicine*, 1972, **65**: 241–2.

71. Perry, J. Uses of the Oxford medical information system in the support of primary medical care. *Colloques I.R.I.A.*, 1974; **1**: 367–8.
72. The Computer Working Party of the Royal College of General Practitioners. *Computers in primary care. Occasional paper* 13. RCGP, London: 1980.
73. Linacre, J. *Evaluation of the Micros for GP scheme (interim report)*. Nottingham Family Practitioner Committee, Nottingham, 1985.
74. Project Evaluation Group. *General practice computing: evaluation of the 'micros for GPs' scheme*. HMSO, London, 1985.
75. Department of Health and Social Security. *Survey of computerised general practices*. NHS Information Technology Branch, London: 1987.
76. Pringle, M. Greeks bearing gifts. *British Medical Journal*, 1987; **295**: 738–9.
77. Technical Working Party of the RCGP/GMSC Joint Computing Group. *The classification of general practice data*. RCGP, London: 1988.
78. Chisholm, J. The Read clinical classification. *British Medical Journal*, 1990; **300**: 1092.
79. Pringle, M. and Harriss, C. *Current Capability of General Practice Computer Software to perform medical audit*. Project report. RCGP, London: 1992.
80. Sweeney, K., Gray, D. Steele, R., and Evans, P. Use of warfarin in non-rheumatic atrial fibrillation: a commentary from general practice. *British Journal of General Practice*, 1995; **45**: 153–158.
81. Howie, J., Hannay, D. and Stevenson, J. *The MacKenzie Report*. Department of General Practice, Edinburgh: 1986.
82. Byrne, P. University departments of general practice and the undergraduate teaching of general practice in the United Kingdom in 1972. *Journal of the Royal College of General Practitioners*, 1973; 23 (Suppl. 1).
83. General Medical Council. *Tomorrow's Doctors*. GMC. London: 1994.
84. Advisory Group on SIFT. *SIFT into the future*. NHS Executive. Leeds: 1995.

2 The NHS reforms

INTRODUCTION

The reforms of the UK National Health Service started in earnest in 1986 with the publication of *Primary health care—an agenda for discussion*,[1] and they continued into the 1990s (Table 2.1). Before considering the changes in detail, it is worth reflecting on the underlying reasons for the reforms, and the extent to which they represent a coherent change. Throughout the early 1980s, the National Health Service was perceived from within to be short of financial resources, and this perception was largely shared by patients. The radical conservative Government of Margaret Thatcher, however, regarded the health service as a major state expenditure over which there was little control. Further, spending on health was rising in real terms through the 1980s, but with each rise in expenditure the louder came the cry for more money. The political liability of the National Health Service was crystallized in the 1987 election campaign when the non-availability of paediatric surgery became a major issue.

Within days of that election, Margaret Thatcher said that she would never again be skewered on the 'health problem'. She chaired an inner group consisting of herself, Nigel Lawson (the Chancellor), John Major (First Secretary to the Treasury), John Moore (Secretary of State for Health and Social Services and incidentally a former First Secretary to the Treasury), and Tony Newton (Minister of Health). When the Department of Health and Social Services was divided, Kenneth Clarke and David Mellor replaced Moore and Newton. Roy Griffiths (the architect of Care in the Community) and John O'Sullivan—a political journalist—also attended regularly.[17] It was this group, with its very strong Treasury bias, that gestated the centre-piece reform, *Working for patients*.[10]

It could be observed that, in one respect, her strategy was successful. In the 1992 election there was a brief skirmish ('the war of Jennifer's ear'), but the health service was not, despite all expectations, a significant issue for the then Prime Minister, John Major. In financial terms, however, it has been less tangibly successful for the Government. Health spending has continued to rise in real terms and as a proportion of Gross Domestic Product, but it is still beneath that of other western countries.

However, the effect of the reforms on those working in the health service has been considerable. The widely reported loss of morale in primary care with a concomitant reduction in applications for vocational training is directly attributed to the 1990 contract[5] and the experience of continual upheaval. The advent of voluntary innovations such as fundholding have been considered divisive while the compulsory aspects of the reforms, for example health promotion clinics, have received widespread criticism. There have been fears concerning the effects of the overall reform package on the doctor–patient relationship, workload, consumerism, and medical independence. While it is too early to

Table 2.1 The principal reports published since the health service reforms started, by main area of focus.

Report	Year published
PRIMARY CARE REFORM	
Neighbourhood nursing—a focus for care	1986[2]
Primary health care—an agenda for discussion	1986[1]
Promoting better health—the government's programme for improving primary health care	1987[3]
General practice in the National Health Service—a new contract	1989[4]
General practice in the National Health Service—the 1990 contract	1989[5]
COMMUNITY CARE/SOCIAL SERVICES REFORM	
Community care—agenda for action	1988[6]
Caring for people	1989[7]
HOSPITAL REFORM	
Hospital medical staffing—achieving a balance	1987[8]
Hospital doctors: training for the future	1993[9]
REFORM OF PRIMARY AND SECONDARY CARE	
Working for patients	1989[10]
Report of the inquiry into London's health service, medical education and research	1992[11]
Managing the new NHS	1993[12]
RESEARCH AND DEVELOPMENT REFORM	
NHS research and development strategy	1991[13]
The Culyer report	1995[14]
STRATEGIC HEALTH SERVICE GOALS	
The health of the nation—a strategy for health in England	1992[15]
The patient's charter	1992[16]

assess the long-term effects of the reforms—and many of the views of today may be seen to be alarmist as the new health service settles in—it is not too soon to pose the question: to what extent were the reforms a coherent, Machiavellian, package designed as complementary pieces in a grand plan for health?

The dates in Table 2.1 suggest the answer. In an overhaul of any organization, the first imperative is to define its overall aim. Only in 1992 with the publication of *The health of the nation*[15] has there been a statement of the objectives of the health service—and these are limited to six key public health issues. The patient's charter[16] has resulted in targets for hospital waiting lists, but it would have been more logical to begin the reforms with a statement of the intent, scope, and standards of health care to be sought (and bought). The second logical area to examine would have been the research and development strategy of the health service, before moving on to relate the structure to the desired processes to achieve the desired outcome. This sounds too cold and clinical for the pragmatic reality of British politics; but the sequencing of the reforms suggests that they were piecemeal and opportunist rather than planned and strategic.

In this chapter, each era of reform—as categorized in Table 2.1—will be briefly discussed. There are great risks in presenting recent history: emotions are still high, memories of events and their significance differ. It is, however, important that a doctor joining general practice has a perspective on the recent past. Each reader is urged, however, to interpret these reforms within their own context.

PRIMARY CARE REFORM

The first hint of the turmoil to come was presented by the Cumberledge report on community nursing.[1] What seemed in prospect like a safe enough area for a committee to examine proved to be dynamite in the hands of Julia (now Lady) Cumberledge, the then chair of South-West Thames Regional Health Authority. For many years there had been a trend for community nurses to be attached to general practices. This led to a dichotomy of loyalty and responsibility—their contact was with the District Health Authority, and their clinical accountability was to nursing managers and the general practice—and some logistic absurdities. A tower block might, for example, be covered by four practices and four teams of district nurses or health visitors. The Cumberledge solution was the formation of neighbourhood nursing teams, geographically rather than practice based. Although it was tried in many areas of the country, it has only been successfully applied in some urban areas, and the inclusion of community nurses in fundholding represents the final demise of the neighbourhood nursing concept.

As is often the case, the headline concept disguised a few ideas which have become central to the primary care reforms. She recommended the introduction of nurse practitioners, an idea still struggling to become established due to repeated delays in legislating for nurse prescribing, and contracts between general practices and community nurse teams. Although the contracts in the internal market and Care in the Community are different from those in the Cumberledge report, this was the first time health contracts had surfaced.

Concurrently the government was focusing on general practice itself. There was a perception of a highly variable level of service between practices, with no clear commitment to preventive care. A discussion document in 1986[2] and the programme published in 1987[3] set out these objectives:

- to make services more responsive to the needs of Government
- to raise standards of care
- to promote health and prevent illness
- to give patients the widest range of choice in obtaining high quality primary care services

- to improve value for money
- to enable clearer priorities to be set for Family Practitioner Services in relation to the rest of the NHS.

It was the perceived role of the Royal College of General Practitioners in these documents that caused it to enter a political limbo for the duration of the reform process (a position from which it is only now recovering). There were discussions between senior college members and the Government on how good practice might be identified and rewarded. The resulting proposal—a 'good practice allowance'—was denounced and derided, and did not reappear in the final programme. It lived on, however, in the spirit and details of the new contract.[4,5]

Indeed the first two primary care papers[2,3] can be seen in retrospect as the setting of the stage for contractual reform. In some ways it is surprising that the profession seemed so unprepared when the first proposals for a new contract were published.[4] The General Medical Services Committee entered into negotiations against a backdrop of protests from general practitioners, and eventually recommended a package that they were able to agree with the Department of Health under Kenneth Clarke. When the profession rejected the agreement at ballot, the Government imposed the new contract anyway.[5] The method of introduction soured any possibility of rational discussion on the merits or demerits of the contract, the main new elements of which were:

a. consumerism

- a shift towards capitation payments
- easier for patients to change doctor, and simplified complaints procedure

b. preventive care

- target payments for cervical cytology and childhood immunizations
- registration medicals
- health promotion clinic payments
- check every three years for non-attenders
- annual health checks on the elderly

c. clinical

- minor surgery payments
- child health surveillance payments

d. education

- postgraduate education allowance
- payment for teaching medical students

e. information

- requirement for annual reports and practice leaflets
- reimbursement of some computer expenses

f. contractual changes

- payment for patients in deprived areas
- retirement by 70
- explicit hours of work and availability
- tightening of arrangements for out-of-hours cover.

From the Government's view, the new contract was a logical part of a process of making general practice more accountable to its patients and its paymaster. Many of the proposals may seem, in that light, quite reasonable. However, the contract was not introduced in a spirit of cooperation through negotiation, and its one-sided genesis was inevitably going to lead to confrontation and acrimony.

The profession has, therefore, still not recovered from the method of introduction—imposition—and from two key features. Firstly, this was the first time that the Government had made explicit what a doctor in the NHS was expected to actually do. Previously, it had been purely an issue of professional accountability—a general practitioner was expected to do what general practitioners normally did. The fracturing of this cosy concept was a key reason for the great distress in general practice throughout 1990.

The second, more important, effect was that general practitioners had to work harder. Some earned more money, while others lost; but all experienced an escalation in their workload. Many practices delegated some of the new tasks, but their administrative workload increased; others tried to accomplish the clinics and targets in addition to their normal clinical load, and often failed to maximize their care and their income.

The last element of 'bad blood' from the new contract resulted from a perception that the Government failed to honour their side of the contract. Kenneth Clarke had stated that he would be delighted if general practitioners responded to the contract so effectively that they dramatically increased their incomes. At the end of the first year, general practice had indeed responded beyond the Government's expectations—and the Government clawed back part of the 'overspend' the next year.

Two issues in the 1990 contract exemplify its shortcomings. The contract was built on a perceived professional consensus and patient opinion in favour of routine screening and case finding in primary care. The evidence for routine checks is, at best, poor and for some of the propositions—regular height recording in adults for example—non-existent. It is quite clear that these proposals were not built upon the burgeoning academic literature concerning screening and primary care, but on reflex assumptions and prejudices.

The second exemplar is the arrangements for postgraduate training. Prior to the 1990 contract there was a system for reimbursement for legitimate expenses incurred from attending postgraduate education, but many general practitioners never claimed. This was seen as evidence that they were not pursuing any education even though in-practice education or journal reading was, by definition, not claimable and many local courses were so low cost as not to justify the effort.

The postgraduate education allowance rewards general practitioners for attendance at approved courses and requires a minimum of five days at a mixture of courses to qualify (for an allowance which was paid from a reduction in seniority payments). This change encouraged a 'bums on seats' approach, rewarding attendance rather than learning and biasing education away from self-directed enquiry back into didactic presentation. The effect of this change was counter to all accepted educational nostrums.

Looked at dispassionately, the new contract can be seen as an attempt to codify and reward the behaviour of the 'best' practices and, to an extent, prepare general practice for the central role that was about to be thrust upon it. It has provoked a remarkable search for evidence with which to question the movement towards screening and prevention, and thus may unwittingly have stimulated the academic base of primary care. However, its content and method of introduction have destroyed a consensus between the profession and the Government in which primary care was being developed in the interests of real quality of patient care.

COMMUNITY CARE / SOCIAL SERVICES REFORM

In 1986, Sir Roy Griffiths was asked by Norman Fowler, the then Secretary of State for Health and Social Services, to examine the community services. This report was prompted by the escalating cost of keeping the sick and elderly in residential and nursing homes—£100m in 1983/84; £850m by 1988/89[7]—and the shift away from long term hospital care.

Griffiths' key recommendation was that the budget for this care should be shifted from social security to the social services—from benefits offices to social workers.[6] The Government responded with its report, *Caring for people*,[7] which was intended for implementation in April 1992, but was delayed until 1993.

The main thrust of *Caring for people* was that patients requiring social care beyond usual health care would be assessed by a social worker who would usually agree a care plan with the practice. This might include the provision of domestic support, extra nursing, or admission to residential or nursing homes.

It was envisaged that much of this extra support will be supplied by contracting private agencies, and that people will be kept in the community—'social security provisions should not, as they do now, provide an incentive in favour of residential and nursing home care'. It is, however, becoming increasingly clear that the resources applied to care in the community were, and are, inadequate to meet the demand. The increasing numbers of elderly patients cannot be adequately accommodated within the budgets and there is under-provision for patients with chronic, severe mental illness. This programme continues to attract robust adverse comment.

HOSPITAL REFORM

The Government approached the secondary care sector with considerably more circumspection. This was partly because the hospitals were traditionally more powerful, militant, and organized than primary care. But it also reflected the fact that the hospitals were 'managed', and changes were passed down through the management structure. The first inkling of the reforms to come was the publication of *Achieving a balance* in 1987,[8] which reviewed the career structure and numbers of all the hospital medical grades. It proposed an increase in consultants alongside a decrease in registrars, and an extension of long-term support grades for doctors not progressing to consultant status. The report was, however, oddly silent on the key issue of junior doctors' hours.

The real reforms in secondary care were to start a little later with *Working for patients*.[10] However the sequel to *Achieving a balance* was the Calman report,[9] published in 1993. This reviewed the numbers of hospital doctors and the training grades, in the light of the reduction in junior doctors' hours and evolving clinical responsibilities. The key recommendation of a shorter training with expansion of the consultant grades is being implemented, as is the assessment of competence before the issuing of a certificate of completion of specialist training.

One key implication for primary care is that every doctor should have general professional training, and that this can be undertaken in primary care. Kenneth Calman, the Chief Medical Officer, is examining the case for reform in primary care staffing and career pathways, and this may further emphasize the potential role of general practice as the main training ground for the health service.

REFORM OF PRIMARY AND SECONDARY CARE

Working for patients[10] was, and is, very closely identified with Mrs Thatcher herself. Indeed she wrote the foreword. It is not one document so much as a whole raft of reforms, most of which were merely hinted at in the original publication. Many of the most radical reforms were, in retrospect, underestimated both in the initial text and in the reaction to it. The main points of the reforms were:

- self-governing hospitals (NHS Trusts)
- the internal market
- the fund-holding scheme for general practices
- indicative prescribing scheme
- medical audit
- creation of Family Health Services Authorities
- an information strategy for the NHS.

Self-governing NHS Trusts

When the National Health Service was formed, the consultants had continued to run the hospitals through Hospital Management Committees with administration being undertaken by a hospital secretary and nursing services being led by the matron. The introduction of managers to the health service through the 1970s and 1980s was partly to professionalize management, partly to free consultants for clinical work and partly to increase accountability. However, the increasing numbers of centrally located managers attracted criticism concerning costs and 'bureaucracy' and a new approach to management was espoused.

In the new internal market (see below) there would be managers who decided what services the NHS should provide and who should provide them—the providers. These services would then be provided, under contract, by hospitals and community groupings called NHS Trusts, each with managers and clinicians. The devolving of responsibility for the delivery of services and the budgets for them to providers—hence the phrase 'purchaser provider split'—was seen as beneficial for a number of reasons: it would empower local management, allow for local contracting, make individual clinicians more accountable, and would facilitate flexibility of provision within contracts.

Hospitals, community units, and ambulance services were encouraged to apply for Trust status with, initially, the remainder continuing to be directly managed by the health authority. In reality very few directly managed units were left by 1994 as Trusts became the standard provider model. Trusts have their own boards, own chief executives, and own management structures. Their autonomy is limited by their contracts and the imperatives of the health service as a whole. Their scope for radical action is, therefore, circumscribed.

The internal market

Trusts would have no logic without an internal market in health care, which was seen by the Government as offering more leverage for better services, value for money, and accountability. In a full blooded internal market, the purchasers of secondary care—the Commissioning Authorities and general practice fundholders (see below)—would contract with NHS Trust Hospitals and Community Trusts, and could choose between them on grounds of cost and quality. Clearly a poor hospital would attract fewer contracts and thus its overheads per patient would rise: it would spiral into bankruptcy and closure. This danger was considered politically unacceptable in the early years of the reforms and thus the internal market in secondary care was restricted from the start through the creation of a 'managed market'. It is still difficult to imagine a major hospital being allowed to call in the receivers, but mergers have been used to disguise closures or downsizing of some Trusts.

Trust hospitals can in theory operate as independent business, attracting patients—and the money that goes with them—from all over the country. In reality the Trusts have not been allowed to operate in a free market. They are obliged to continue with a full range of services and the central purchasers, the District Health Authorities, continue to buy patient care along traditional patterns. There has been pressure against extra-contractual referrals by nonfundholder general practitioners—that is, referrals outside the local district. The internal market has exposed the paucity of information available concerning numbers of patients treated, the costs of each treatment and the size of waiting lists. Practices had no idea of the possible demand for secondary care, nor of the numbers of patients waiting. Not one element of the information jigsaw puzzle required for an internal market was in place and in many areas continue to be missing.

The internal market was not just seen as affecting secondary care and community service providers. General practices are providers of primary care services and for them the internal market was expected to improve services. A strong purchaser in the guise of the Family Health Services Authority (now merging into the Commissioning Authorities) was thought likely to insist on high standards, augmented by patients who would support the functioning of the internal market by preferentially registering with 'good' practices.

In fact, the General Practice Contract is determined in central negotiations between the General Medical Services Committee and the Department of Health, negating local leverage; and Family Health Service Authorities have never been encouraged to enforce the terms of the contract rigorously. Further, patients have not proved to be particularly powerful in the market place—they have not been rewarding good practices and punishing the bad through mass migrations between practices.

Further evidence of the dilution of the internal market could be seen in the *Health of the Nation* initiative.[15] Although laudable as a strategic statement of the goals of the health service, it sets priorities nationally when, in theory, the purchasers should set them locally. It is this conflict between autonomy and market forces, and the need to offer a cohesive service throughout the country, that lies at the heart of the internal market dilemma. However, the moves towards an internal market have raised the collective consciousness of the health service concerning costs, value for money, cash limits, and rationing. This is seen most clearly in the transformation of general practices into purchasing fundholders.

The fundholding scheme for general practices

Fundholding, as a radical dimension of the internal market, was dismissed in the early years as a peripheral sideshow. The idea of general practitioners effectively buying secondary care services was dismissed as an irrelevance. At this stage of the reforms, with over half of patients registered with a fundholding practice, it could be argued that the internal market has been powered by fundholders who have prevented cosy cartels developing between hospital trusts and health authorities. As total purchasing practices (fundholders who purchase almost all external services for their patients) develop, fundholding may become the predominant model for the purchasing of secondary care and community services. However, political and managerial imperatives may roll back the influence of fundholders in the next few years.

In essence, standard fundholding practices negotiate a fund from their Commissioning Authority (before April 1994 with their Regional Health Authority, and up to April 1996 with the Family Health Services Authority) to cover much of the non-acute hospital care for their patients, the drugs prescribed in the practice, practice staffing, and community nursing. They then negotiate contracts with hospitals and community units and pay for the services they use outside the practice. Total purchasing practices also include acute care in their fund while community fundholders cover fewer areas of care than the standard ones.

Hospital contracts can be block (one fee for unlimited services—for example for pathology or radiology), cost and volume (a fee for a number of cases), or cost per case (each referral is paid for individually). A practice can save money by withdrawing patients from routine follow-up, reducing unnecessary referrals or reducing the cost of referrals (for example by holding consultant clinics in the practice), reducing the numbers of procedures done on their patients, or by 'shopping around'. Savings can be spent on improved patient care in the practice, including improvements to premises.

Many fundholding practices have indeed saved considerable money from their funds, usually from the hospital section. This means that money is flowing from the secondary care sector into primary care. The restrictions in the internal market inhibit hospitals from making up the shortfall through full blooded competition. It also means that practices are making important investment decisions that affect the shape of the health service—is it better to employ a physiotherapist or do three hip replacements? These are difficult and complex health economic decisions for which general practitioners have never been prepared, and their piecemeal nature mitigates against coherent policy initiatives for the public's health.

Perhaps the most revealing consequence of fundholding has been the discovery of transaction costs. Of course transaction costs—the cost of the bureaucracy behind patient movements through the health service—have always existed but the internal market, and specifically fundholding, has made them explicit. In fundholding practices, fund administration absorbs between 2 per cent and 3 per cent of the fund—money which previously was available for patient care. Only if comparable savings in the cost of patient care were demonstrated could the transaction costs in the fund be justified, but even then they cannot be justified in the health service as a whole—money 'saved' by fundholders in their secondary care budget is lost to the hospitals where, of course, transaction costs have also increased.

On the positive side, the advent of fundholding has had a significant effect on the quality of service offered by many hospitals and their consultants; there is a palpably improved commitment to patient care both in the consumerist 'hotel' and in the clinical aspects. Fundholders have increased their practice management skills and have often improved the primary care services to their patients.

Indicative prescribing scheme

All general practitioners have been involved in the indicative prescribing scheme in which they have been set theoretical budgets for their drug costs, and have been monitored against these amounts. The flaws have become clear. The scheme has no teeth, and overspending practices face no sanctions. The annual increase has been inadequate, and virtually all practices have exceeded their funds. Lastly, the doctors have no real ownership of their budgets—the Family Health Service Authority notifies them of its size. For these reasons the indicative prescribing scheme has not been a success, but it has stimulated thinking about prescribing costs and improved the information systems available to monitor them.

Medical audit

The proposals for medical audit in *Working for patients* were widely welcomed. In hospitals, Medical Audit Committees have been formed, audit facilitators appointed, and many computers brought. Cynics would point out that not much auditing has actually resulted. The appointment of Medical Audit Advisory Groups (MAAGs) in each Family Health Service Authority area appears to have uncovered, or possibly promoted, a considerable level of audit activity in primary care. Nearly half of all general practitioners take part in auditing, although, as discussed in the previous chapter, evidence that auditing activity improves patient care is hard to come by. The key characteristics of the MAAG scheme is that medical audit is still voluntary and professionally led, but it is resourced and supported administratively so that the cultural climate is substantially in its favour.

The Family Health Services Authorities

One aspect of *Working for patients* which has had a considerable impact on general practice was the creation of Family Health Services Authorities, although their life has been a short one. Before 1989, the Family Practitioner Committees were concerned with 'pay and rations' but were not primarily involved in standard setting, contract monitoring, or cost effectiveness. They were accountable directly to the Department of Health.

Working for Patients created new authorities, accountable to Regional Health Authorities (RHAs)—now regional offices of the NHS Executive. These Family Health Service Authorities (FHSAs), with a slim management group, employed independent medical advisers, nursing advisers, and public health advisers. They were increasingly concerned with cost-effective prescribing, quality of minor surgery, health promotion strategies, and so on.

On April 1 1996, the FHSAs merged with the District Health Authorities to create combined Commissioning Authorities. The extent to which the primary care agenda can remain paramount within combined authorities remains to be seen, but many fear that the high tide mark of general practice influence within the health service has already been reached.

Information strategy

The last element to the reforms concerns the information strategy. It is clear that the Department of Health is committed to creating an infrastructure on which information technology can flourish. It has purchased the Read Codes for example, created the NHS Centre for Coding and Classification to support them, and is funding the Clinical Terms Project to extend them. An NHS network is being built up, and protocols for its use established. A Minimum System Specification for general practice has been undertaken, and general practice computing is being reviewed and supported.

The *Working for patients* initiative represents a cultural shift in the health service of substantial proportions. The power and position of general practice has been appreciably enhanced as has its responsibilities and workload. It heralded a sustained period of change which was unsettling and challenging. However, *Working for patients* was not the final major reform, leaving mere tinkering to occur at the margins. This was illustrated by the Tomlinson report on health care in London.[11] The proposal to merge eight London medical schools into four received wide comment, but a large section of the report concerned a strategy for improving primary care in London, including the augmentation of its resources. It is too early to say how the London reforms will work and what long-term effects they will have; it can be asserted, however, that they illustrate the continuing anger and frustration engendered by structural changes and the new thinking—primary care is the jewel in the health service. The clearest evidence for this is in the rhetoric of a 'primary care led NHS'.[18] While it is often not exactly clear what speakers mean by this term, the philosophy of enhancing primary care must be welcomed, albeit with the caution reserved for possible poisoned chalices.

As already mentioned, the continuing pressure on government spending combined with the decentralizing forces within the health service eventually has led to yet another health authority reorganization.[12] The NHS Executive, which has moved to Leeds, has eight regional offices which replaced the 14 Regional Health Authorities and the bodies which supervise trust hospitals, which were called outposts. Under these regional offices, which will supervise the performance of purchasers and providers but will not intervene in day to day management, will be between 80 and 90 Commissioning Authorities, which will replace the Family Health Services Authorities and the District Health Authorities.

There is a logic and attraction to this simplification of the management structure, and it complements the new functions of the health service. The case for amalgamation includes the realization that, with the movement of hospital management out of District Health Authorities, the need to reduce managers in health authorities has decreased; and that commissioning—the long-term planning for health service purchasing—involves both primary and secondary care. If the long-term ambition of enhancing primary care at the expense of secondary care is to be realized, then unitary authorities with one fund are essential.

However, it must be observed that primary care will lose its advocate within the structure and may find that its case is less easily heard. The size of the secondary care budget so clearly outweighs that of primary care that the emphasis of policy making may unduly reflect hospital issues. The reduction in the regional role may remove the one possible counter-weight. Further, the new regions may not support the primary care regional structures with the same alacrity as the old ones.

RESEARCH AND DEVELOPMENT REFORM

With the appointment of Professor Michael Peckham as the director of NHS research and development, the Government was belatedly acknowledging that such a substantial organization as the NHS requires an emphasis on R. and D. His strategy[13] signalled a sea-change: increased resources and no longer a reliance on the research community to set the agenda. The next few years will see an increased emphasis on research issues being identified at Department of Health and Regional level, and funds being put behind the answering of those questions. This will inevitably involve more research into the delivery of health care in preference to pure clinical research, and this may well increase opportunities for primary care research. In 1995, the Culyer report[14] proposed all R. and D. funding should be explicit and should arise from a top slicing of all health service funds. This process will involve health authorities in identifying all expenditure on R. and D. and contributing additional money to the central and regional research programmes.

STRATEGIC HEALTH SERVICE GOALS

The last elements in the reform puzzle are *The health of the nation*[15] and *The patients' charter*.[16] That the National Health Service, after over forty years, should start to describe its outcomes in epidemiological and patient terms is probably best described as 'better late than never'.

The Health of the nation concept went out to consultation and was then published as a programme with specific targets in (examples are given):

- Coronary heart disease and stroke
  - to reduce deaths in people under 65 by 40 per cent by year 2000
  - to reduce smoking to 20 per cent of adults by year 2000
- Cancers
  - to reduce the breast cancer death rate by 25 per cent by year 2000
  - to reduce invasive cancer of cervix by 20 per cent by year 2000
  - to reduce lung cancer in men by 30 per cent by 2010
- Mental illness
  - to reduce suicide rate by 15 per cent by year 2000
- HIV/AIDS and sexual health
  - to reduce gonorrhoea by 20 per cent by 1995
  - to reduce under 16s conceptions by 50 per cent by year 2000
- Accidents
  - to reduce deaths from accidents in childhood by 33 per cent by 2005

Many of these targets are merely extrapolations of current trends and might well be achieved without new efforts. The next set of key areas are likely to include asthma and diabetes, both important areas of general practice work.

The patients' charter, and its primary care version, comes direct from John Major's Citizens' Charter. Its effect on the health service, and general practice in particular, is difficult to gauge, but it may link with medical audit and fundholding to provide a platform for demonstrating the high standards of most general practice. For many general practitioners it is seen, however, as a cause of the increase in militant consumerism and thus increased consultation rates (including night visits), increased complaints (many spurious), and an increasing tendency for patients to expect more than the health service can reasonably deliver.

CONCLUSIONS

These have been turbulent times, and the greatest storms may yet be to come. But at this point in the reform process it can be seen that most of the changes have had positive as well as negative aspects, and that they have one common theme—the well-being of general practice is central to the future of the health service. To appreciate the intricacies of the reforms requires wide reading, including the original documents; and for every reform there are opposing opinions. This brief review has tried to highlight the main changes and their effects from a primary care perspective.

REFERENCES

1. Community Nursing Review (Chair: Julia Cumberledge). *Neighbourhood nursing—a focus for care.* London: HMSO, 1986.
2. Secretaries of State for Social Services, Wales, Northern Ireland, and Scotland. *Primary health care—an agenda for discussion.* London: HMSO, 1986.
3. Secretaries of State for Social Services, Wales, Northern Ireland, and Scotland. *Promoting better health—the government's programme for improving primary health care.* London: HMSO, 1987.
4. Department of Health and the Welsh Office. *General practice in the National Health Service—a new contract.* London: Department of Health, 1989.
5. Department of Health and the Welsh Office. *General practice in the National Health Service—the 1990 contract.* London: Department of Health, 1989.
6. Griffiths, R. *Community care—agenda for action.* London: HMSO, 1988.
7. Secretaries of State for Health, Social Security, Wales, Northern Ireland, and Scotland. *Caring for people.* London: HMSO, 1989.
8. The UK Departments of Health, the Joint Consultants' Committee, and Chairmen of Regional Health Authorities. *Hospital medical staffing—achieving a balance.* London: Department of Health, 1987.
9. Department of Health Working Group on Specialist Medical Training (Chairman: Kenneth Calman). *Hospital doctors: training for the future.* London: Department of Health, 1993.

10. Secretaries of State for Health, Wales, Northern Ireland, and Scotland. *Working for patients*. London: HMSO, 1989.
11. Tomlinson, B. *Report of the inquiry into London's health service, medical education and research*. London: HMSO, 1992.
12. Department of Health. *Managing the new NHS*. London: Department of Health, 1993.
13. NHS Management Executive. *NHS research and development strategy*. London: Department of Health, 1991.
14. Research and Development Task Force (Chair: Professor A. Culyer). *Supporting research and development in the NHS*. HMSO, London: 1994.
15. Secretary of State for Health. *The health of the nation—a strategy for health in England*. London: HMSO, 1992.
16. Department of Health. *The patient's charter*. London: Department of Health, 1992.
17. Lawson, N. *The view from No. 11*, pp. 612–4. London: Bantam Press, 1992.
18. NHS Executive. *Developing purchasing and GP fundholding* (EL(94)79). NHSE, Leeds, 1994.

3 Career choices

INTRODUCTION

In broad terms there are twice as many general practitioners as consultants in all specialties combined—in 1989, 29556 general practitioners compared to 16452 consultants.[1] While 15 per cent of consultants are women, a quarter of British general practitioners are women and the proportion is rising quickly. This chapter looks at the system that leads 30000 of the brightest graduates to choose a career in general practice. In doing so it will look at careers guidance for undergraduates and house officers; the route to entry into general practice; and the work experience of groups of principals.

UNDERGRADUATES

Entry to medical school is heavily dependent on success in the A-level examinations. Although many universities still interview applicants, acceptance on the medical course is largely determined by the achievement of the 'right grades'. This has risen from three 'C' grades in the 1960s to two 'A's and a 'B' in the 1990s.

It has to be questioned, however, whether exam success is a valid criterion of entry into medicine. Patients clearly prize doctors who listen and take time and who consult in adequate premises,[2] with clinical expertise being largely taken for granted. The literature does not report patients praising their doctor's intelligence or ability to pass exams. While clinical competence requires a degree of intellectual facility, it is clearly not the prime determinant. The emphasis on 'A'-levels, and the increasing grades expected, result from the operation of crude market forces. There is a gross excess of applicants for medicine—20 for every place; higher than any other course[3]—and there is only one cheap and readily available measure that can be used to distinguish between them. However, it introduces biases into selection, including racial discrimination.[4, 5]

Once at medical school, students have little exposure to careers guidance. Over half of the medical schools in England and Wales have an annual careers fair organized by the British Medical Association which usually involves members of each speciality offering advice as to how their career path is structured. Although this is highly laudable, it falls far short of answering individual questions and matching strengths and weaknesses to career options. No medical school offers psychometric testing and individual guidance before students make decisions that will effect forty years or more of their working lives. It is of interest to observe that applicants for managerial jobs in the National Health Service authorities now usually have a pre-interview psychometric assessment to determine their suitability. Although, of course, psychometric testing alone would never be sufficient—it should be supplemented by personal interview and assessment—insufficient care is taken over the selection of undergraduates and their subsequent career choices.

It appears that most medical students choose a career on the basis of role models and their exposure to that area of work as undergraduates. While general practice employs two thirds of all fully qualified doctors and undertakes nine out of every ten consultations, it accounts for between 2 per cent and 4 per cent of curricular time. The traditional one month general practice attachment has, however, one significant advantage. It is the only part of the undergraduate course where the student experiences one-to-one teaching, and the intensity of the personal experience offers students a unique insight into how one branch of the profession works.

Since the General Medical Council published *Tomorrow's doctors*[6] medical schools have been reviewing their curricula, sometimes with dramatic effects. In essence, the changes involve a reduction in factual knowledge by one third, an emphasis on developing life-long skills for medicine (such as critical thinking, keeping up to date, clinical skills, communication skills, management,[7] and problem solving), early clinical contact, and increased community based teaching.[8-10]

The most radical of the new curricula involve a significant element of student led learning.[11] Students are presented with a topic, for example cervical cytology, and are expected to define a number of questions. In this case the questions might relate to the clinical presentation and epidemiology of cervical cancer; the history of screening; the practical aspects of screening; its relationship to the characteristics of screening programmes; and the effectiveness of the programme. Individual students will work on different questions, reporting back to the group on their findings.

A movement away from passive education in a lecture theatre towards active learning is to be welcomed. It will however require increased access to knowledge based, computer assisted learning (CAL) packages, and tutors with sophisticated teaching skills. Already the requirement for medical schools to define what they aim to teach has been beneficial and if the new curricula can be maintained and can fulfil their promise, then the medical students of tomorrow will be better equipped for the challenge of general practice.

THE EARLY YEARS

It is not surprising therefore that 69 per cent of doctors change their career choice in the ten years after qualification. In their survey of doctors qualifying in 1974 and 1977,[12] Parkhouse and Ellis showed that, while 31 per cent stayed with their original career choice, 30 per cent changed their choice once and 9 per cent changed it four or more times. At qualification 35 per cent chose general practice, with this increasing to 48 per cent six years later. The main reasons given by general practitioners for their career choice were aptitude and ability, domestic circumstances, previous experience of general practice, and promotion prospects/difficulties. They did not rate the financial motive highly.

Another study, this time in the 1980s, showed that general practice was the initial career choice on qualifying of 39 per cent of men and 53 per cent of women.[13] Even on these rising percentages—albeit slowly—up to a third of all general practitioners have made an initial career choice in another field. Many will have migrated to primary care as a preference—their original choice having proved less attractive than at first imagined—but for a significant number the choice of general practice will be forced.

When vocational training became mandatory by law in 1981 it was hoped by many established general practitioners that this would mark the end of general practice being seen, as Lord Moran described it, as the refuge for 'those who had fallen off the consultant ladder'. However, the recent dramatic decline in applications for vocational training schemes has demonstrated that general practice is increasingly seen as an unattractive career choice due to the up-heavals of the new contract, stress, and workload. These dissatisfactions have been crystallized in the debate about out-of-hours care with many young doctors preferring a less onerous commitment than the traditional 24 hour model.

VOCATIONAL TRAINING

By the time a doctor has joined a general practice vocational training scheme, he or she has usually expressed a career choice for general practice. However, one study showed that 2 per cent of men and 11 per cent of women go on to work, after vocational training, in other specialities, and nearly one third of women ex-vocational trainees surveyed were not working as a general practitioner.[14] Only 6 per cent of these were on maternity leave or caring for young children. A more recent study showed that 13 per cent of men ex-trainees and 29 per cent of women were not working in general practice, and that 3 per cent of men and 25 per cent of women had never been a principal in general practice at any time.[15] It appears therefore that increasing numbers of doctors are not entering long-term general practice after vocational training.

The experience during the hospital-based part of vocational training varies but most trainees experience obstetrics and gynaecology, accident and emergency, and paediatrics[16] (Table 3.1). Considering the decline in *intra-partum* care and the emphasis on psychological medicine in general practice, it has to be asked if these hospital posts represent the correct balance for the future.

WOMEN GENERAL PRACTITIONERS

Women are in a special position in medicine. They now represent just over half the entrants to medical schools[3] where they usually study full time. Nearly half

Table 3.1 The hospital post experience submitted for completion of vocational training (per cent of doctors)[16]

	Per cent of doctors		
Hospital post	1985	1988	1990
Obstetrics/gynaecology	86	89	94
Accident and emergency/			
general surgery	66	70	74
Paediatrics	57	60	62
General medicine	46	46	45
Geriatric medicine	36	41	42
Psychiatry	36	40	41

marry other doctors[17] and five years after leaving a vocational training scheme one in five were unmarried (compared to one in twenty men).[14] In the early years of their medical career most have marital and family responsibilities to juggle alongside their medicine, and as we have seen they have a greater preference for a career in general practice.[11]

The reasons for the preference for general practice include the shorter time until finishing the training grades, a perception that completion of training is more predictable, and the availability of part-time working. Indeed practices have in recent years perceived a female partner to be an asset, a necessary asset in the consumerist market place of the reformed NHS.

The attraction of female partners can be directly attributed to the rise in patient expectation for choice. When female patients were asked if they had a preference of sex of doctor, over 80 per cent had no preference when they had a general health problem. But over half would prefer a female doctor or nurse when they have a women's health problem or require an intimate examination.[18] The road to partnership is, however, fraught. Firth-Cozens showed that 46 per cent of female junior house officers had scores on the general health questionaire and the symptom checklist for depression that were above those for diagnosing clinical depression.[19] The explanations included overwork, the effects of work on their personal lives, relationships with consultants, sexual harassment at work, and prejudice from patients.

The number of women on vocational training schemes has been rising. In 1981 just over a third of vocational trainees were women, while nearly half are women in the early 1990s. Female graduates are more likely to have periods of unemployment: 4 in 10 are unemployed for over three months compared to only 1 in 10 male graduates.[20] By the time they have established themselves in a career, 56 per cent will be in general practice, 31 per cent in hospital medicine, 4 per cent in community medicine, and 2 per cent in academia.[21]

Misconceptions concerning the workload of women general practitioners date from early studies which lumped women working part time with those working full time and compared their workload to predominantly full time male general practitioners. In fact, full time women partners do an equal workload to full time men,[22] although their caseload is slightly different. They see more women patients, especially in their child bearing years, and have more consultations for cervical cytology, contraception, and breast disorders.[23] They are half as likely compared to men, however, to be involved in teaching or research.[15]

While full time women general practitioners do an equal share of on call,[22] overall only three quarters do weekend cover (compared to over 90 per cent of men) and women spend on average two hours less consulting per week.[24] They are also less likely to be single handed or to work in deprived inner city areas.

Women doctors working part time, on the other hand, are often exploited by the partnership. While they average 76 per cent of a full time partner's workload, two thirds are on a partnership share of less than half a full timer.[25] While a third do no out of hours work, two thirds do more out of hours than their profit share would suggest. They also may be less involved in partnership finances and practice management.

PART TIME WORK

Most part time general practitioners are female and up to 40 per cent of females opt for part time work,[17,20] One recent study showed that 45 per cent of female and 6 per cent of male general practitioners either were, or wished to, work part time.[26] This compares to only 3 per cent of male general practitioners working part time. In the hospital service part time posts are usually not training posts and are therefore often described as 'dead end' jobs.[17] In contrast, part time principals in general practice may be at the peak of their discipline and are valued team members.

Part time general practitioners have either a personal commitment to the practice which is less than full time or they offer a full time service in combination with one other doctor—a job share arrangement. What evidence there is[27] suggests that job share partners gain equivalent patient satisfaction to full time partners, but this is a relatively new form of working which will need evaluation with time.

Only 2 per cent of women are part time because they split their working with other jobs.[21] They are more usually part time due to family commitments. The Statement of Fees and Allowances acknowledges two part time levels of commitment which influence the proportion of the basic practice allowance that the practice receives. The practice agreement may, however, state a different degree of commitment and this determines the partnership share—the share of the partnership profits—that the part time partner receives. In addition, there is the actual workload of the part time partner and this often substantially exceeds the partnership share. A job sharing arrangement can be seen as a protection against some of the inequalities experienced by part time partners. If two doctors are offering a full time service to the practice they have a strong claim to a full share in the partnership profits. And since one or other is always present, the pressure for one to increase their commitment is reduced.

If a general practitioner does not work full time, the possibilities for establishing a portfolio of occupations opens up. For many women doctors a key occupation is that of mother; but for many part time doctors their general practice is combined with a clinical assistantship at a hospital, a teaching or research post, a job in industrial or occupational health, or a role in management. Many of these options are described in Chapter 5.

ETHNIC MINORITY DOCTORS

It is a sad fact that ethnic minority doctors often find it much more difficult to succeed at every stage of their career. A common explanation centres on the supposed inadequacies of medical training, particularly in the New Commonwealth. However, non-Europeans who graduate from British medical schools find career progression equally difficult. After overcoming the discrimination evident in medical school entry procedures,[4,5] doctors from ethnic minorities encounter problems with jobs. When applying for a first senior house officer post, 14 per cent of European graduates of British medical schools reported having made 10 or more unsuccessful applications, compared to 22 per cent of ethnic minority graduates of British medical schools.[11] The ethnic minority graduates were more likely to be unemployed, with 8 per cent reporting unemployment of over three months, compared to 3 per cent of their European contemporaries. Problems in entering partnerships have resulted in a higher proportion of single handed doctors being from ethnic minorities and their contribution to primary care in inner city and deprived areas is noticeably higher. One of the key challenges which British general practice faces is to acknowledge the in-built prejudices in the health service; to educate themselves and their colleagues to counter it; and to integrate isolated ethnic minority doctors into the mainstream of general practice.

CONCLUSIONS

General practice occupies the centre stage of the health service. It is, however, the first choice of career of only one third of medical students and this may be a reflection of the low level of career guidance given in medical schools. It may, however, be a symptom of a basic lack of attraction in our discipline, which might explain the falling numbers of applications for vocational training. Two groups of general practitioners have special problems. Women have fewer opportunities, more unemployment and finally end up in less satisfactory posts than men. Doctors from ethnic minorities confront prejudice and reduced opportunities.

REFERENCES

1. Medical Manpower and Education Division of Department of Health. Medical and dental staffing prospects in the NHS in England and Wales 1989. *Health Trends*, 1990; **3**: 96–103.
2. Cartwright, A. and Anderson R. *General practice revisited*. London: Tavistock Publications, 1981.
3. UCCA: *The thirtieth report, 1991–2*. Cheltenhan: UCCA, 1993.
4. McManus, M., Richards, P., Winder, B., Sproston, K., and Styles, V. Medical school applicants from ethnic minority groups: identifying if and when they are disadvantaged. British Medical Journal. 1995; **310**: 496–500.
5. Esmail, A., Nelson, P., Primarolo, D., and Toma, T. Acceptance into medical school, and racial discrimination. *British Medical Journal*, 1995; **310**: 501–2.
6. General Medical Council. *Tomorrow's doctors*. GMC, London: 1994.
7. Fairhurst, K., Stanley, I., and Griffiths, C. Should medical students learn more about management? *British Journal of General Practice*, 1995; **45**: 2–3.
8. Field, J. and Kinmonth, A.-L. Learning medicine in the community. *British Medical Journal*, 1995; **310**: 343–4.
9. Robinson, L., Spencer, J., and Jones, R. Contribution of academic departments of general practice to undergraduate teaching, and the plans for curriculum development. *British Journal of General Practice*, 1994, **44**: 489–91.
10. Foldevi, M. Undergraduate medical students' rating of clerkship in general practice. *Family Practice*, 1995; **12**: 207–13.
11. Bligh, J. Problem based, small group learning. *British Medical Journal*, 1995; **311**: 342–3.
12. Parkhouse, J. and Ellin, D. Reasons for doctors' career choice and change of choice. *British Medical Journal*, 1988; **296**: 1651–3.
13. McKeigue, P., Richards, J., and Richards, P. Effects of discrimination by sex and race on the early careers of British medical graduates during 1981–7. *British Medical Journal*, 1990; **301**: 961–4.
14. Osler, K. Employment experiences of vocationally trained doctors. *British Medical Journal*, 1991; **303**: 762–4.
15. Johnson, N., Hasler, J., Mant, D., Randall, T., Jones. L., and Yudkin, P. General practice careers: changing experience of men and women vocational trainees between 1974 and 1989. *British Journal of General Practice*, 1993; **43**: 141–5.
16. Styles, W. Training experience of doctors certified for general practice in 1985–90. *British Journal of General Practice*, 1991; **41**: 488–91.
17. Allen, I. *Doctors and their careers*. London: Policy Studies Institute, 1988.
18. Nichols, S. Women's preferences for sex of doctor: a postal survey. *Journal of the Royal College of General Practitioners*, 1987; **37**: 540–3.
19. Firth-Cozens, J. Sources of stress in women junior house officers. *British Medical Journal*, 1990; **301**: 89–91.
20. Rhodes, P. Medical women in the middle: family or career? *Health Trends*, 1990; **22**: 33–6.

21. Wakeford, R. and Warren, V. Women doctors' career choice and commitment to medicine: implications for general practice. *Journal of the Royal College of General Practitioners*, 1989; **39**: 91–5.
22. Hooper, J. Full time women general practitioners—an invaluable asset. *Journal of the Royal College of General Practitioners*, 1989; **39**: 289–91.
23. Cooke, M. and Ronalds, C. Women doctors in urban general practice: the patients. *British Medical Journal*, 1985; **290**: 753–5.
24. Cooke, M. and Ronalds, C. Women doctors in urban general practice: the doctors. *British Medical Journal*, 1985; **290**: 755–8.
25. Hooper, J., Millar, J., Schofield, P., and Ward, G. Part-time women general practitioners—workload and remuneration. *Journal of the Royal College of General Practitioners*, 1989; **39**: 400–3.
26. Breadlow, R., Cheung, K., and Styles, W. Factors influencing the career choices of general practitioner trainees in North West Thames Regional Health Authority. *British Journal of General Practice*, 1993; **43**: 449–52.
27. Nicol, E. Job sharing in general practice. *British Medical Journal*, 1987; **295**: 888–90.

4 The topography of general practice

INTRODUCTION

Every general practitioner works within a landscape—a social, business, and health topography. This landscape is defined by the contracts that each practitioner has with themselves, their colleagues, their patients, society, the profession, and the health service. Within these contracts their workload is defined by patient demand, disease, and the other services provided. This chapter looks at the contracts that circumscribe our work and the work that we actually do. Of necessity this has to be superficial; in some respects there is a world of difference between practices in inner city Liverpool and a village in the Home Counties; between a dispensing practice in the Highlands of Scotland and a practice based in a wealthy London suburb. However, there is also much that they share, and this chapter explores that common territory in the topography of general practice.

CONTRACTS

Every principal in general practice has a contract with the National Health Service and usually a contract—a partnership agreement—with the practice. There are additionally a professional 'contract' which is policed by the General Medical Council; a 'contract' with the registered patients which has been most recently codified in the Patient's Charter for Primary Care; and finally a legal 'contract' under which the doctor can be held to account for negligence.

The contract with the National Health Service[1] implicitly sets out the independent contractor status of the general practitioner. Unlike independent contractors in other areas of business, the general practitioner has an indefinite contract which only routinely terminates at the age of seventy; has access to an index linked pension fund; and, until recently, had no quality criteria attached to the contracted work. The 1990 contract[2] was imposed on a reluctant profession and it started a process under which the general practice contract became more normal for an 'independent contractor'. The purchaser, in this case the Department of Health, began to stipulate certain performance criteria which were to be rewarded—the achievement of targets for immunization and cervical cytology and attendance at postgraduate education, for example. (These performance criteria may not be those valued by the contractor, but they are valued sufficiently by the purchaser to be codified in contract.)

This is not the place for a detailed description of the current general practice contract—there are other documents which can be consulted.[1,3] Suffice to say, it is made up of direct reimbursements, capitation payments, target payment, items of service and activity payments, and incentive payments such as deprivation payments. While a doctor can decide not to offer many services, such as child development surveillance, the core services are not optional and failure to supply them is a breach of the terms and conditions of service.

If a patient complains to the Family Health Services Authority about a doctor the case is considered to see if it applies to the core services. Complaints about diagnostic acumen are not usually accepted, but an alleged failure to visit a patient would be. If the complaint is judged to be relevant and it is in time, the doctor is asked to respond to the allegation before a hearing occurs. If the doctor is found to have been in breach, a fine can be imposed. This takes the form of the Family Health Services Authority withholding payments. The numbers of complaints from patients are increasing at present which probably reflects a growing awareness of the complaints process rather than a decline in the standards of general practice; but a formal complaint still only occurs once for every 60 000 consultations.

Changes in the state contract to look out for in the future will include contracts with the practice not the individual, short-term contracts renewable on adequate performance, and a defined range of services that are a minimum requirement. The liability of a doctor for the behaviour of other doctors acting on his or her behalf—locums, trainees or deputizing services—will cease and the arrangements for out-of-hours care will be revised. Recertification at intervals of, say, five years will be introduced.

The contract between a general practitioner and the partnership is a different animal altogether. The partnership agreement sets out the legal framework for the conduct of the practice and covers the handling and division of money, sickness, holidays and sabbaticals, dissolution, assets such as premises, and partner conduct. A happy practice should only need to refer to its partnership agreement when a new partner joins the practice. However, if things go wrong, a partnership agreement is the rock on which solutions are built.

Traditionally, the General Medical Council has been concerned with professional misconduct, sickness without insight such as alcoholism, and gross incompetence. Such a safety net captures only the most extreme form of behaviour and cannot address, for example, poor clinical skills. Recently, the General Medical Council has been moving towards a counselling service for illness and a monitoring service for incompetence.[4] Both may increase its role in protecting the public from poor standards, but without re-certification it is likely to be only scratching the surface.

The contracts with patients may be without sanctions in the technical sense, but they have a powerful emotional imperative. Some patients expect to know what services are available to them and they expect those services to be high quality. If they are not, they can vote with their feet by leaving a practice, which they seldom do, or they can make their displeasure known. Such an appeal to the professionalism of the doctors can be very successful in changing the standards of care. More usually the patients keep quiet and become resigned to poor care.

The other side of the contract with patients is the one that states how the patients should use the service of the practice. Few practices have actually written this down although the Patient's Charter[5] explicitly encourages them to do so. In time it is likely that the contract with patients will become more explicit, with practices defining unacceptable patient behaviour at the same time as they define the standards patients should expect.

Recently, some patients have been grouping together to increase their power in their implicit contracts with practices. One manifestation is patient participation groups which are often created with the support of the partners to change the balance of communication and to help the practice to be more responsive.[6] These groups have, however, often become vehicles for fund-raising and supporting the practice rather than serious organizations for improving patient care.

Another type of patient group is that centred on a disease or condition. The British Diabetic Association, for example, has drawn up protocols which state the care a diabetic should expect from a general practitioner.[7] This move is laudable but does increase the patient's role in the care contract. In time many patient groups may join in and it is to be hoped that they do not unreasonably raise expectations, but remain mindful of the realities of care.

There has been an increased fear of litigation with the American experience much quoted.[8] However, in the United States the litigant has only to prove harm, here he or she must also prove negligence. Certainly, every practising doctor must be a member of a medical defence insurance group but the risk of being sued is still, thankfully, small. There has been much controversy surrounding the concept of no fault compensation. If a patient is found, for example, on recovering from an anaesthetic to be hemiplegic, the cause is crucial. If it was due to negligence by an anaesthetist a court may award a six figure sum. If it was due to a chance embolic event, the patient has no compensation. This situation clearly denies equity and encourages litigation. The solution proposed by some—and implemented in, for example, Scandinavia and New Zealand—is to compensate everybody who comes to harm in the process of or as a result of medical care and leave the punishment of negligence to the medical profession or the courts. In New Zealand, this concept has been extended to include compensation of all injuries but the abuse of this system by patients and doctors alike has placed it in jeopardy.

These, then, are the contracts that define the environment in which we work. There is also, of course, the most important contract of all—the contract that a professional holds with him or herself, the professional conscience—which underpins the whole health enterprise. It is this contract that is manifest through honesty, the pursuit of quality, innovation, and excellence. Any changes to the other contracts that erode the professional imperative will be detrimental for patient care.

WORKLOAD

General practice accounted for £5 billion of expenditure in 1993, one sixth of

Table 4.1 Practice size—number of partners per practice in 1992

Number of partners	Per cent of practices
1	10
2	14
3	19
4	18
5	17
6 +	22

the total for the National Health Service. Of this, 60 per cent was payment for drugs prescribed in primary care, so general medical services themselves cost only one pound in fifteen. The average patient had 7.5 prescriptions per year at an average cost of £7 per prescription. The average general practitioner prescribed drugs costing £105 000 in a year.

Ninety per cent of practices are partnerships, with nearly a quarter having six or more partners (Table 4.1). While there is no consensus concerning the ideal list size, a survey of general practitioner attitudes showed that if lower list sizes were obtained, most doctors would increase their length of consultation, their consulting rate per patient, and their home visiting, but would expect a drop in the overall time spent at work.[9] The General Medical Services Committee has an historical aim of an average list size of 1 700 throughout the United Kingdom.[10]

The fourth national study of *Morbidity statistics from general practice*, published in 1995 but covering 1991 and 1992, showed that 78 per cent of patients consult their general practitioner in a year, averaging 3.8 consultations per year[11] (up from 3.5 consultations per year ten years earlier[18]). By comparison, Fry and Dillane have demonstrated a consultation rate in their practice of 3.5 per patient per year in the mid-1950s, which has fallen to 2.3 by the mid-1980s.[12] A comparison with consultation rates found in the *General household survey 1992*[13] for different age groups is given in Table 4.2.

Certain groups of patients are known to have higher consulting rates than

Table 4.2 Mean number of consultations per year with general practitioners for age and sex groups from the 4th *Morbidity statistics from general practice* (MSGP4)[11] and the *General household survey* (GHS)[13]

Age group	MSGP4		GHS	
	Men	Women	Men	Women
0–4	5.1	4.8	6.8	6.5
5–14	2.3	2.6	2.8	2.9
15–44	2.1	4.2	2.4	4.8
45–64	3.0	4.0	3.5	4.9
65–74	4.2	4.6	4.8	5.4
75 +	5.6	6.3	6.9	5.4

others. Patients with a lower social class consult more[14, 15] as do those living in council accommodation and those from ethnic minorities.[14, 16, 17] While overall 78 per cent of patients consult their general practitioner, there are large age and sex variations—98 per cent of all children under 5 consult in one year, for example.[11] Of episodes seen by general practitioners 46 per cent were classified as 'trivial', 40 per cent 'intermediate' and 14 per cent serious.

Home visits are decreasing[12] with one study showing a 71 per cent decrease in visits to patients aged less than 65 in the years 1977 to 1989.[19] This study also highlighted the fact that three quarters of visits are requested by patients aged 65 or over, and that this is the section of the population set to increase in size: home visiting might therefore become more common again. Each takes longer than a surgery consultation—an average of 16 minutes in Sheffield[20] for example.

The hours that general practitioners work is a repetitive source of contention. In one recent survey, the average general practitioner worked 40.6 hours per week on delivering general medical services, 4.5 hours on other medical activity, and 17.8 hours on out-of-hours work. These doctors were working 63 hours a week[20] which was the same as a year earlier before the introduction of the new contract. However, the new contract's introduction in 1990 was associated with doctors spending two hours more per week in the surgery, offering more clinics, employing more staff, and increasing their list size.[21]

Table 4.3 shows the broad categories of consulting in the fourth Morbidity Statistics from General Practice,[11] and Table 4.4 shows the rate of chronic disease per 10 000 patients found in one rural practice. Geographical differences in morbidity presenting to a general practice have been found. In the North of

Table 4.3 Consulting rates per 10 000 patients per year for chapters in the International Classification of Diseases[11]

ICD chapters	Consultations
Infectious and parasitic diseases	1399
Neoplasms	239
Endocrine	377
Mental disorders	728
Diseases of nervous system and sense organs	1732
Diseases of the circulatory system	931
Diseases of the respiratory system	3070
Diseases of digestive system	866
Diseases of genito-urinary system	1133
Diseases of skin	1455
Diseases of musculo-skeletal system	1522
Injury and poisoning	1390
Signs, symptoms and ill defined	1510
Procedures	3348
Other	271

Table 4.4 The prevalence of six chronic diseases in a rural population expressed as a rate per 10 000 patients adjusted to the European standard population

Diagnosis	Rate per 10 000 population
Asthma	645
Hypertension	596
Ischaemic Heart Disease	404
Diabetes	168
Dementia	64
Glaucoma	61

England there are more consultations for respiratory disease other than asthma, cardiovascular disease, and cerebrovascular disease; but fewer consultations for diabetes. In the South, Midlands, and Wales there are more consultations for hypertension, and in the Midlands and Wales fewer consultations for cervical cytology.[22] There are marked differences between even such large areas as Family Health Service Authorities as Table 4.5 shows.[23] The great variations between practices are eloquently illustrated by the 20 fold variation in referral rates.[24]

Clearly general practitioners vary in their views on what they should be delivering to their patients. There seems a clear consensus that internal medicine is definitely part of general practice, but less consensus concerning psycho-social problems and technical issues, such as toe-nail removal, gynaecology, and orthopaedics.[25] Younger general practitioners do more pathology tests, more referrals and more cervical cytology, but prescribe less.[26] Rurality appears to have no real influence on workload, including, surprisingly, home visiting rates.[27]

STRESS IN GENERAL PRACTICE

It might be thought that a career in general practice was as close to perfection

Table 4.5 The range between the highest and lowest Family Health Service Authorities (FHSAs) on a range of performance indicators[23]

Performance indicator	Highest FHSA	Lowest FHSA
Drug cost per patient	£62.35	£30.71
Health promotion payments per patient	£2.70	£0.20
% practices achieving 70% immunization	100%	27%
% practices achieving 60% cervical cytology	100%	38%
Minor surgery sessions paid per GP	12.1	0.8

as man could get. It is a well paid job with a high level of autonomy and responsibility. General practitioners are held in high esteem by society and there is a generous pension scheme to which he or she can look forward. Indeed it is the freedom to choose the method of working, responsibility, and variety that give most job satisfaction to general practitioners, while the rate of pay and the hours of work create dissatisfaction. The greatest stress in a doctor's day comes from interruptions, emotional involvement, administration, and the home-work interface. It appears that the major stresses are social, not medical.[28] This has been confirmed by general practitioners who kept mood diaries. Their mood was lowest when they were hassled, under time pressure, or had domestic dissatisfaction; their mood was highest when working efficiently and to time.[29] A repeated survey showed that 'doctors experienced more stress, less job satisfaction, and poorer health in 1990 then in 1987'.[30]

Patient-centred doctors experience more stress—they described over a third of their consultations as stressful compared to one in ten for their doctor centred colleagues—as do all general practitioners when patients are booked too frequently for their style of consulting.[31] Longer consultations are more likely to be described as satisfactory (37 per cent) than short ones (28 per cent) and are therefore seen to be less stressful.[32] One very stressful aspect of general practice is the constant threat of patient aggression. In one major study, 91 per cent of general practitioners had experienced verbal abuse, 18 per cent attempted injury and 11 per cent actual injury.[33]

It seems that stress is increasing and one explanation appears possible. In the early days of the National Health Service general practice had enough flexibility and slack to absorb many new tasks. It has coped with vocational training and the move to preventive care, increased staffing, and computerization. However, general practice has now become saturated with tasks and additional tasks, such as those encapsulated in the new contract, cannot be easily assimilated. These new tasks include the care for an increasing range of clinical conditions. Few patients with chronic disease are now referred to hospital and those that are referred are seen in outpatients for fewer visits. Day surgery and early discharge after more substantial surgery places greater onus on primary care services; and the advent of minor surgery, endoscopy, vasectomy, and other procedures in general practice increases the movement of services from secondary to primary care.

While this migration of clinical workload has been occurring, general practices have also been accumulating a new range of managerial responsibilities, with many fundholding practices having budgets of over £2m. Commissioning Authorities are courting general practitioners to assist with their purchasing decisions; Medical Audit Advisory Groups are expecting more and more sophisticated audits; and practice teams require more and more meetings. . . .

The concurrent increase in consumerism has placed a greater expectation on doctors in their additional tasks as reflected in the greatly increased rates of out-of-hours calls.[34] One symptom of this conflict is the high level of violence endured by general practitioners, and another is the problems with recruitment and retention. Applications for practice vacancies are at an historic low and many general practitioners are retiring early. It may be that the perception of stress expressed by many general practitioners is a symptom of a system about to collapse—or it might just be a reaction to imposed change. Only time will tell.

REFERENCES

1. Department of Health. *Statement of fees and allowances*. London: Department of Health, 1994.
2. Department of Health and the Welsh Office. *General practice in the National Health Service—a new contract*. London: Department of Health, 1989.
3. Chisholm, J. *Making sense of the new contract*. Oxford: Radcliffe Medical Press, 1990.
4. General Medical Council. *Proposals for new performance procedures: a consultation paper*. London: GMC, 1992.
5. Department of Health. *The patient's charter*. London: Department of Health, 1992.
6. Pritchard, P. *Patient participation in general practice*. Occasional paper 17. London: Royal College of General Practitioners, 1981.
7. British Diabetic Association. *Guidelines for the management of diabetes*. London: BDA, 1990.
8. Medical Defence Union. *Annual report*. London: MDU, 1993.
9. Butler, J. and Calnan, M. List sizes and use of time in general practice. *British Medical Journal*, 1987; **295**: 1383–6.
10. General Medical Services Committee. *General practice: a British success*. London: British Medical Association, 1983.
11. Royal College of General Practitioners, The Office of Population Censuses and Surveys, and the Department of Health. *Morbidity Statistics from General Practice, fourth national study 1991–1992*. London: OPCS, 1995.
12. Fry, J. and Dillane, J. Workload in a general practice 1950–85. *Journal of the Royal College of General Practitioners*, 1986; **36**: 403–4.
13. Office of Population Censuses and Surveys Social Survey Division. *The general household survey 1992*. London: HMSO, 1994.
14. Balarajan, R., Yuen, P., and Machin, D. Deprivation and general practitioner workload. *British Medical Journal*, 1992; **304**: 529–34.
15. Cook, D., Morris, J., Walker, M., and Shaper, A. Consultation rates among middle aged men in general practice over three years. *British Medical Journal*, 1990; **301**: 647–50.
16. Gilliam, S. J., Jarman, B., White, P., and Law, R. Ethnic differences in consulting rates in urban general practice. *British Medical Journal*, 1989; **299**: 953–7.
17. Balarajan, R., Yuen, P., and Raleigh, V. Ethnic differences in general practitioner consultations. *British Medical Journal*, 1989; **299**: 958–60.
18. Royal College of General Practitioners, Office of Population Censuses and Surveys and Department of Health and Social Security. *Morbidity statistics from general practice—third national study*. London: HMSO, 1983.
19. Beale, N. Daily home visiting in one general practice: a longitudinal study of patient-initiated workload. *British Journal of General Practice*, 1991; **41**: 16–18.
20. Hannay, D., Usherwood, T., and Platts, M. Workload of general practitioners before and after the new contract. *British Medical Journal*, 1992; **304**: 615–8.
21. Hannay, D., Usherwood, T., and Platts, M. Practice organisation before and after the new contract: a survey of general practices in Sheffield. *British Journal of General Practice*, 1992; **42**: 517–20.

22. Fleming, D. and Crombie, D. Geographical variations in persons consulting rates in general practice in England and Wales. *Health Trends*, 1989; **21**: 51–5.
23. Audit Commission. *Practices make perfect: the role of the FHSAs*. Local Government report no. 10. London: HMSO, 1993.
24. Wilkin, D. and Smith, A. Explaining variation in general practitioner referrals to hospital. *Family Practice*, 1987; **4**: 160–9.
25. Whitfield, M. and Bucks, R. General practitioners responsibilities to their patients. *British Medical Journal*, 1988; **297**: 398–400.
26. Armstrong, D. and Griffin, G. Patterns of work in general practice in the Bromley health district. *Journal of the Royal College of General Practitioners*, 1987; **37**: 264–6.
27. Fearn, R. Norfolk general practice: a comparison of rural and urban doctors. *Journal of the Royal College of General Practitioners*, 1988; **38**: 270–3.
28. Makin, P., Rout, U., and Cooper, C. Job satisfaction and occupational stress among general practitioners—a pilot study. *Journal of the Royal College of General Practitioners*, 1988; **38**: 303–6.
29. Rankin, H., Serieys, N., and Elliot-Binns, C. Determinants of mood in general practitioners. *British Medical Journal*, 1987; **294**: 618–20.
30. Sutherland, V. and Cooper, C. Job stress, satisfaction, and mental health among general practitioners before and after introduction of new contract. *British Medical Journal*, 1992; **304**: 1545–8.
31. Howie, J., Hopton, J., Heaney, D., and Porter, A. Attitudes to medical care, the organisation of work and stress among general practitioners. *British Journal of General Practice*, 1992; **42**: 181–5.
32. Heaney, D., Howie, J., and Porter, A. Factors influencing waiting times and consultation times in general practice. *British Journal of General Practice*, 1991; **41**: 315–9.
33. D'Urso, P. and Hobbs, R. Aggression and the general practitioner. *British Medical Journal*, 1989; **298**: 97–8.
34. Heath, I. General practice at night. *British Medical Journal*, 1995; **311**: 466.

5 Opportunities in general practice

INTRODUCTION

One of the initial benefits, but potential long-term drawbacks, of the choice of a life in general practice is the absence of a career progression. At 27 or 28, a doctor can leave vocational training and join a practice for perhaps as long as 40 years. Within a few years of joining that practice, the doctor will be a full partner on maximum earnings. It is true that the challenge of clinical improvement is never ending and seems particularly daunting in the early years; and that, as we have seen, practices are constantly reacting to changes in their environment and in their internal relationships. But many general practitioners experience a feeling in their mid-thirties that their professional life is becoming too routine, that the main challenges of primary care have been confronted and that an element of control has been established. This is often the time when young general practitioners begin to look around for new opportunities and challenges. This chapter will outline some of these.

THE CLINICAL ENDEAVOUR

The most universal challenge is the one within the consultation—to deliver high quality care to the patients. Although this may seem self-evident, many general practitioners place continuing medical education low on their priorities, and we appear to esteem medico-political leaders above good clinicians. This is because clinical excellence is hidden from immediate view in the confidentiality of the consulting room, and also because much good care is proactive and it is, therefore, difficult to demonstrate.

A good clinician keeps up-to-date through imaginative, intelligent use of lectures, seminars, the journals, and distance learning. An invaluable source is, however, immediate colleagues. Discussions in which clinical behaviour is debated can be powerful facilitators towards quality. Such discussions might centre around the setting of standards in one area and their auditing; a journal club; a review of evidence; or a case discussion. For many general practitioners a rigorous examination of individual cases offers a powerful stimulus to quality.[1-5] To be effective it must be conducted among those you trust in a spirit of improvement, not blame allocation. Case discussions often result in congratulations and celebration of good care—something which is all too rare in our professional lives. The discussion might end in a decision to undertake a conventional audit or, sometimes, immediate change in clinical policy or habits is required.

Once established, many general practitioners look for a way to demonstrate to their peers that a high quality of care is being achieved. This aspiration has been met by the arrival of Fellowship by Assessment of the Royal College of General

Practitioners.[6] This is a system for self-nomination for Fellowship by those College members who can demonstrate that they meet every one of the published criteria. These include that the applicant must have been a member of the College for five years and have been a principal for five years. This does not, of course, exclude a new entrant into general practice from getting the criteria and using them as a guide or template in developing their practice and their personal skills.

All those who pass the membership examination are told about Fellowship by Assessment, and anyone interested can contact the Royal College of General Practitioners. Once a general practitioner believes that he or she will be ready to apply within the next year, they sign an 'intention to apply' which freezes the existing criteria (they are updated annually) for one year. When they apply within that year, the criteria at the time of indicating their intention will be those against which they are assessed. Faculty advisers help applicants to understand the precise requirements of each criteria and the applicant gathers the documentation, including a videotape of twelve consecutive consultations. The assessment takes the form of a visit to the practice by three Fellows who examine the equipment, facilities and systems, and talk to the applicant's colleagues. Success results in a recommendation for the award of Fellowship.

In the first six years of Fellowship by Assessment there were seventy success-ful applicants, and the number is growing geometrically. It is envisaged that, in time, success in the MRCGP examination will be seen as a milestone—certainly a significant milestone—on the road to the demonstration of quality of general practice through Fellowship by Assessment.

EDUCATIONAL DEVELOPMENT

The Royal College of General Practitioners has long been campaigning[7] for the first years in practice to have a structured educational content. All too often a doctor completes vocational training, hopefully crowning it with success in the MRCGP, and then regards formal education as complete. Educational develop-ment is then left to the pot luck of the courses, lectures, and seminars that come through the post. One future alternative would be to incorporate the concept of higher professional training into the early years in practice. This might involve protected time for professional education with clear objectives within the early years. Although this idea has substantial intellectual support, political support has so far been scanty.

Many young general practitioners respond, however, by embarking on their own structured education. This can be through portfolio learning, which is a needs based personal educational programme. Others do it through Master of Science or similar courses.[8] Many university departments of general practice and public health medicine run M.Sc. courses. The market for taught higher degree courses is competitive with the supply of places often exceeding the number of potential applicants able and willing to commit the time and money involved. This has helped to ensure that the standard of these courses has been maintained at a high level. They come in two broad groups.

One group of courses is aimed at general practitioners and primary care professionals. In addition to a broad emphasis on scientific method, epidemiology, and health care organization, these concentrate on adding an academic dimension to the primary care task. A graduate should have a much clearer vision of the political, social, economic, and clinical context in which they work, and to have completed a research project which has enhanced and demonstrated scientific skills. The second group tend to be more specialized, but attract many general practitioners. Some offer a specialized M.Sc. degree, such as one in sports medicine. Others focus on related skills areas, such as a Master of Public Health degree. Some general practitioners undertake courses for training in counselling, psychosexual or otherwise, while others join Balint groups.[9]

Almost all these options require perseverance and stamina, and they also often require time off to be negotiated with the practice. Many courses charge significant fees, although some sponsorship may be available, and require evening and weekend working—they are therefore a strain on family life. For these reasons only a minority of general practitioners choose this route, but those that do often have the commitment to be the professional leaders of the future.

BECOMING A VOCATIONAL TRAINER

For most young principals their immediate role model in general practice is their vocational trainer. While others may include a parent, their childhood general practitioner, a partner in the training practice, or a partner in their new practice: for most the trainer–registrar relationship is seminal. If the trainer was a contented, independent, fulfilled person and the relationship was warm and supportive, then it is only natural that the young principal should aspire to be a trainer to replicate the experience. And trainers are, of course, intended to be good role models. They are chosen for their personal, clinical, and organizational skills and they work in the better organized practices. They have regular trainers' workshops to maintain their enthusiasm and motivation, and they go on trainers' courses to maintain and develop their teaching skills.

However, a first problem can be that one in five young principals join practices that are already undertaking vocational training. If the existing trainer is relatively young and enjoying the task and if the practice is too small to have two registrars, the route to being a vocational trainer may be blocked. In these circumstances many young partners start by covering for the trainer when he or she is away on holiday, and then work towards sharing the training responsibility. The end result may be that alternative registrars are allocated between two trainers. However, this is often not possible.

A second problem is that the standards required of the practice itself are usually clear and uncompromising. Each region has its own standards, which can be obtained from the Regional Adviser (see below) and which cover such areas as the medical records, use of deputizing services, and access to a primary health care team. There is often a stipulation that the registrar must have their own consulting room as well as access to an adequate medical library within the practice. In a co-operative practice that is committed to improving its standards these problems are usually surmountable; if the prospective trainer does not have such a high level of mutual support, reaching the standards may present real difficulties.

The third problem can be personal qualification. Many schemes now insist that every trainer should have the MRCGP examination. For some prospective trainers tentative feelers are rebuffed because the Course Organizers (see below) do not perceive that the applicant has the right personality or skills for vocational training. One solution to this is for the aspiring trainer to ask for, and accept, honest advice from his or her own trainer or some other mentor.

If a young principal can succeed in becoming a vocational trainer this often is, in itself, sufficient to offer the intellectual edge which many are seeking. The camaraderie between trainers, the questioning from the registrar, the constant needs to justify and evaluate—all these offer an emotional and intellectual framework for personal development. Vocational trainers are paid a fee and their practice gains a working doctor, although one who cannot and must not work to the same workload as full partners. For many practices the attraction of vocational training is that the task can be 'fitted into the routine day'—teaching can occur before and after surgeries; tutorials can be squeezed into lunch times. Nowadays, however, it is clear that training really does require a commitment on behalf of the practice to offer quality teaching time in which the trainer and the registrar are allowed uninterrupted regular, protected sessions. If practices are not prepared to fulfil their side of the training bargain, it is unlikely that they will continue training for long.

BECOMING AN EXAMINER

One exclusive club that is worth aspiring to is that of the examiners for the Membership of the Royal College of General Practitioners. The examiners are usually trainers or course organizers with obliging and co-operative practices and seeking an extra challenge—it involves about fifteen days away from the practice every year.

The examiners enjoy the company of a select and exciting group of their peers and share with them an important task. Many examiners undertake it for between five and ten years before moving on, but almost all current and former examiners would rate it as one of their most rewarding activities. Any general practitioners who are confident in their organizational and clinical skills, with the support of an efficient caring practice, and who wish to consider becoming an examiner should contact the Royal College of General Practitioners.

THE POSTGRADUATE STRUCTURE

There are four recognized jobs within the postgraduate structure—Course Organiser, GP Tutor, Associate Regional Adviser, and Regional Adviser—but first a few words about the structure's context. Regional Advisers are, as of 1995, university appointees and they are therefore clearly within an educational frame rather than a health service frame. The Regional Adviser is responsible to the Postgraduate Dean, and is accountable to a regional post-graduate committee, whose title varies from region to region. It is anticipated that in 1996 the Postgraduate Deans—so far, never from primary care—will become health service posts within the structure of the regional office, although the precise details of the new Regional Adviser contract are still obscure.

The Regional Adviser is responsible for leading all postgraduate education, including vocational training, in the region, and has, therefore, a role in appointing and supervising Course Organisers and, through them, Vocational Trainers. This aspect of their work is examined in regular visits from representatives of the Joint Committee on Postgraduate Training for General Practice—a statutory body on which the Royal College of General Practitioners and the General Medical Services Committee have equal representation. So, the Regional Adviser with a number of Associate Regional Advisers is responsible for monitoring vocational training, including posts in hospital and general practice, and for ensuring that the educational potentials are maximized. He or she is also responsible for administering the educational approval system for the Postgraduate Educational Allowance, and often for the Retainer Scheme.

Within this structure there is little formal accountability to the profession itself, and none at present to the Department of Health—hence the change of the Postgraduate Deans from university to Civil Service posts. A successful postgraduate team relies, however, on maintaining credibility with and support from general practice itself.

Course Organisers have the responsibility for organizing and supervising the vocational training schemes, and on bigger schemes this role is split between several Course Organisers. They work alongside GP Tutors (who are confusingly called 'Course Organisers' in some regions) who are based in postgraduate medical education centres and who work at developing primary care through continuing medical education for established principals. Course Organisers and GP Tutors are paid for sessions at the consultant rate of pay, but their commitment can be more onerous than that of trainers. They usually have to spend their course organizing time away from the practice and their flexibility is limited. Traditionally, Course Organisers were former trainers, but increasingly prospective trainers and those with wider educational ambitions take up these posts.

One route for those with ambitions is up the structure from Course Organiser to Associate Regional Adviser or a Regional Adviser. Regional Advisers represent the top of the postgraduate field for general practitioners at present (although it is to be hoped that Postgraduate Dean posts will be open to general practitioners) and in that sense are equivalent to the head of the undergraduate department of general practice. Indeed, in one region, the Regional Adviser is also Professor in the Postgraduate Department of General Practice and in another has a personal chair.

General practice is the only discipline in which there is a dichotomy between the undergraduate and postgraduate teachers. While this has arisen for understandable historical reasons, it has no logic and no clear benefit. Increasingly the two sides are coming closer,[10] but a consistent, countrywide union still seems a long way off. If amalgamation is to be achieved, the different cultures, administrations, and regulatory frameworks will need to be reconciled.

Regional Advisers and their Associates are highly skilled pedagogues who have developed a wide interest in medical education. Many take an active part in developing and researching aspects of medical education and they have considerable influence in regional educational committees. There is at least one Regional Adviser in every NHS Region, with more than one where there are multiple medical schools—for example in the Trent Region where there are Regional Advisers in Leicester, Nottingham, and Sheffield.

UNDERGRADUATE TEACHING

There is an accelerating trend for medical schools' curricula to be based in the community. The contrast with the 1960s, when general practice was, at best, a one week option, could not be greater. In many medical schools the students now visit practices and are taught by general practitioners in every year of the course, including the pre-clinical years.

The criteria for becoming an undergraduate teacher are sometimes less formal and stringent that those for vocational training, although they are identical in other parts of the country. Two key ingredients are sought—enthusiasm and proximity to the medical school, although in some areas, notably Wessex, the latter is not regarded as important. Many undergraduate teaching practices also undertake vocational training and this teaching culture in the practice makes them attractive to undergraduate departments. Teaching students can be challenging and enjoyable. They ask questions about the core of our business, about the very essence of primary care, and this helps teachers to freshen their approach. They undertake audits and they test out the information systems. They represent an opportunity for a practice to influence the future generation of doctors and to attract the brightest and the best into primary care.

Students cannot, however, lighten the workload of a practice—indeed by sitting in on consultations they slow things down. They often come for short periods, perhaps a month, and then just as they are becoming familiar they are replaced by another eager face. They can, moreover, through their enquiring minds, lead to a much larger time commitment than the notional expectation. The best way to judge this form of teaching is to talk to undergraduate teachers and their partners—and their practice managers. It is likely that all will emphasise the positive and negative aspects almost equally, but they will rate something indefinable as being vitally important—involvement in the academic endeavour of primary care.

THE ACADEMIC ENDEAVOUR

The teachers of undergraduates represent one part of the academic endeavour, much of which happens outside university departments. Indeed, many vocational trainers contribute significantly. For the purposes of this section, however, the academic endeavour will be interpreted in a restricted sense. When a doctor decides to pursue knowledge and academic excellence there are established paths to follow. Some, however, choose to make their own paths and do so successfully. The most obvious of the established paths' is through the career structure of academic departments of general practice.

Usually, general practitioners start by teaching students in their practices and thus mature a relationship with the department, but this is not necessarily the case. Many lecturers start by replying to advertisements in the refereed journals. The status of Part Time Lecturer or Tutor is often given to teachers of undergraduates, but the title of Lecturer infers a greater commitment. Lecturers teach undergraduates in the core curriculum as well as in their general practice attachments; they assist in departmental administration; they may undertake postgraduate teaching; and they are expected to do research. It is protected time for research that marks this breed out as they pursue the holy grail of medical academia, the Doctorate.

An MD (or DM in some universities) is awarded for a thesis, often with a viva, which offers a new dimension of knowledge for the discipline. This usually involved submitting a coherent body of research in one particular area which explores new ground and which, by its comprehensive nature, offers a new understanding. For some this is a lifetime's work, especially if done whilst a full time general practitioner. For those with protected research time and access to research grants, it will take a minimum of three years. It is, however, not beyond the capacity of any general practitioner and, alongside Fellowship by Assessment, should be one of the main targets for the intellectually restless young principal.

Once an MD has been acquired, then the Senior Lecturer and Professorial posts beckon. Some are content to continue researching in the lecturer grade, but equally the career ladder proves irresistible for others. Senior Lecturers are often half time or less in general practice and they carry a significant part of the organizational workload in the department. Every medical school has a Professor of General Practice except for two, and these have academic departments. Professors are responsible for organizing the general practice input into the undergraduate curricula, and for supporting and undertaking research. They have, however, wider responsibilities to their medical schools, the university and primary care as a whole.

In all this, research must be emphasized as one of the noble, if under-rewarded, pursuits for a young principal to consider. If any discipline is to thrive it must have a corpus of knowledge which it nurtures, owns, and develops; it must have skills that are defined, recognized, and unique; and it must have its own political respectability to further its case. Research contributes to all three and it is an essential part of the infra-structure of a vibrant discipline. Research also offers the greater vision, the higher academic task, that can give meaning to a life in one general practice. Not every general practitioner could, or would wish to undertake research, but for those that do, it offers a stimulus and enjoyment which is unsurpassed. While research may lead to a higher degree, to a chair in general practice, or recognition from your peers, much research is done for the sheer enjoyment of finding out, for the exhilaration of the intellectual chase, and as such is a justification in itself.

MEDICAL POLITICS

In its loosest sense this includes work for the Local Medical Committee, the local faculty of the Royal College of General Practitioners, the General Medical Services Committee, the Council of the Royal College of General Practitioners, and the General Medical Council. These are all routes to fame and notoriety; assisting the profession or being rejected by it; furthering primary care or becoming frustrated. Medical politics are for those with an interest for big issues and their small corners, and may require considerable personal, family, and practice commitment for little return. However, for the breed that are attracted by debate, emotion, and the challenge of issues, the enjoyment is compensation enough.

CLINICAL AVENUES

Once established in practice, many young principals find themselves under pressure to use their medical skills to contribute to the income of the practice; some seek out other applications for their clinical skills. The possibilities are enormous, and they cannot be adequately enumerated or described here. They include industrial medicine with many large companies employing sessional doctors; private medical companies, with BUPA, for example, employing many doctors to undertake their routine examinations; family planning clinics and termination counselling services; working in prisons, with all but the largest prisons using local general practitioners for sessional work and on-call cover; aviation or diving medicals which require special training and accreditation; insurance medicals; and clinical assistantships.

Clinical assistant posts offer an opportunity to join a specialist team for a limited number of sessions every week, seeing a case-mix that radically differs from the patients seen in a general practice surgery, and developing a clinical expertise that can be of considerable use to the practice. A special skill in dermatology or sigmoidoscopy, as examples, can contribute to the range of services and their quality available on the practice premises. Some doctors rotate regularly through hospital departments, augmenting their clinical skills as they go.

On the negative side, a young doctor has to be careful that the clinical assistantship offers real training opportunities and does not only involve seeing 'follow-ups'; that the time spent on such commitments does not detract from the care they offer in practice, especially at times of pressure such as holidays; and that the practice does not become so dependent on the income that giving up the appointment would be problematic.

NHS MANAGEMENT

There is a need for experienced general practitioners to become involved with the health authorities as medical advisers and, increasingly, officers. Many general practitioners start by joining committees that advise on commissioning, share views on fundholding, or are part of the statutory complaints procedure. A few become interested in offering advice to the officers in health authorities or Trust (especially community trusts).

The role of Independent Medical Adviser to the Family Health Services Authority was created and made mandatory in 1990 as a method for ensuring that Family Health Service Authority officers had access to a general practitioner who was not also on the Local Medical Committee. The role has varied from a full-time post to a few hours a week, and there is an association of medical advisers which represents their interests. The work can be interesting—discovering how the health service actually works can be a revelation—but it is also demanding and stressful. As Family Health Service Authorities are merged into health commissions the long term role of Independent Medical Advisers is unclear.

Most health authorities now have a manager responsible for general practice —a director of primary care, primary care development, or equivalent—and some of these now have clinical backgrounds, including general practitioners. Some general practitioners are doing Master of Public Health courses and are joining departments of public health in health commissions to offer primary care expertise. In time, general practitioners will start appearing in the ranks of the chief executives.

Beyond medical advising (and even then it is difficult), these options involve a career change, away from clinical care in general practice into NHS management. Such moves are not for the faint-hearted and those making them are often trying to leave practice as much as to arrive at a new opportunity.

CONCLUSIONS

General practice can be an end in itself, and for many indubitably it is. One way of demonstrating that general practice itself has been achieved to the highest standard is by taking Fellowship by Assessment. For many doctors, however, there are other challenges and excitements to add lustre to a career in general practice. These include education, academia, or medical politics, but may also involve clinical posts outside the practice, journalism, business, or health service administration. As a general practitioner, provided your practice will support you, the world is your oyster.

REFERENCES

1. Pringle, M., Bradley, C., Carmichael, C., Wallis, H., and Moore, A. *Significant event auditing*. Occasional paper 70. London: Royal College of General Practitioners, 1995.
2. Hussain, L. and Redmond, A. Are pre-hospital deaths from accidental injury preventable? *British Medical Journal*, 1994; **308**: 1077–80.
3. Foldevi, M., Somansson, G., and Trell, E. Problem-based medical education in general practice: experience from Linkoping, Sweden. *British Journal of General Practice*, 1994; **44**: 473–6.
4. Pringle, M. and Bradley, C. Significant event auditing: a user's guide. *Audit Trends*, 1994; **2**: 20–3.
5. Robinson, L., Stacy, R., Spencer, J., and Bhopal, R. Use of facilitated case discussions for significant event auditing, *British Medical Journal*, 1995: **311**: 315–18.
6. Royal College of General Practitioners. *Fellowship by assessment*, Occasional paper 50. London: RCGP, 1990.
7. Royal College of General Practitioners. *The front line of the health service*. London: RCGP, 1987.
8. Smith, L. Higher professional training in general practice: provision of master's degree courses in the United Kingdom in 1993. *British Medical Journal*, 1994; **308**: 1679–82.
9. Balint, M. *The doctor, his patient and the illness*. London: Pitman Medical, 1957.
10. Bain, J., Scott, R., and Snadden, D. Integrating undergraduate and postgraduate education in general practice: experience in Tayside. *British Medical Journal*, 1995; **310**: 1577–79.

6 The future of primary care

INTRODUCTION

A chapter on the future of primary care can be seen as, and maybe is, an indulgence. It is, however, one way of pointing out the current trends and examining the possibilities. Although many of the predictions in this chapter will never be realized, their possibility may alert the reader to the tensions and options that, in the authors' opinion, they can expect during their career in primary care. This chapter is, therefore, a survey of those trends that can already be identified with a commentary that attempts to interpret their possible effects.

THE DISCIPLINE

Primary care can, and often is, viewed as either the other disciplines (medicine, gynaecology, dermatology, and so on) practised outside hospitals, or as what is left behind when all the others have defined their territory—the discipline of miscellaneous affairs. While general practitioners have understood for years that they have a special corpus of knowledge which they deploy with special skills, this has not been well appreciated outside our closed circles.

As the call for evidence based medicine becomes louder, we will need to define for others the knowledge and skills which we call our own. An earlier generation saw this need at the start of vocational training with the *Future general practitioner*,[1] and we are now attempting the same in our time with *The nature of general medical practice*.[2] We need to start with a consensus on what we do—the content of our discipline—before we can move forward.

We will then need to define our knowledge base,[3,4] identifying those aspects that are truly ours and those that are borrowed—perhaps incorrectly—from other disciplines. For example Sweeney and colleagues have shown how our 'evidence' on treating patients with atrial fibrillation is based on heavily selected groups in a hospital setting and they speculate that such evidence might not hold good for the undifferentiated population in primary care.[5]

The next decade confronts us, therefore, with a formidable task. We need to persuade ourselves first, and then others, of the nature of our discipline and we need to explore its knowledge base more rigorously than has previously been accomplished. Alongside this endeavour we will be developing our skills and showing how they have been especially refined for the delivery of care in a community setting. This agenda for the discipline as a whole must, however, run concurrently with a number of identifiable agendas which we must respond to—not least that of our patients.

PATIENTS

One of the defining changes of the fourth quarter of the twentieth century has been consumerism and the empowerment of, in this context, patients. This trend has not yet run its full course and seems to have potential for significantly influencing primary care in the future. In the absence of any formal controls over decisions made in fundholding practices, patient groups are likely to enter the accountability vacuum. The passive, friendly patient participation groups of today are likely to be replaced by more assertive, better informed groups which are prepared to monitor the health needs and services of the population. A sensitive practice will soon have a management board which commissions the health care for its population, and this board will have representation from patients and staff. Its decisions will be public and will be based on logic and facts. The patient representative will be reporting to the practice patients and will be expected to express their views. The level of communication between doctors, nurses, and practice managers and their patients as a whole will, hopefully, improve. Newsletters will become common; charters will be common-place and will be updated regularly; standards will be audited and the results shared with the public.

Perhaps the most interesting result will be that practices will define the precise outcomes that they wish to achieve. These will be in the form of clinical control (for example glycosylated haemoglobin in diabetics), events they wish to reduce (such as strokes or accidents), life-styles they wish to encourage (reducing adult smoking), and secondary care they wish to buy. The choices in making such decisions will be overt and sophisticated and will reflect not just the health needs of their population but also the health priorities.

In Oregon, since 1988, the public has been asked to select the core services that the health service, as funded from the state, should provide. The debate has been overtly about rationing and prioritizing—in a world of finite resources should reversal of sterilization be offered in preference to hip replacements? Of 688 diseases, the consultative exercise identified 568 to be paid for from Medicaid since the scheme's introduction in 1994, and every year further diseases are de-listed. The NHS, unlike the American health service, does not fact the same stark choices in rationing, but some health authorities have decided that cosmetic surgery, fertility therapy, and reversal of sterilization should not be available as part of 'normal' services. As these rationing choices become more common, patient involvement—probably to a lesser extent than that tried in Oregon—will become equally common.

Such a patient orientated world will involve a loss of power and autonomy for general practitioners, but this is precisely the trend that has dominated the last few decades. Patient power will be sufficiently strong to ensure that the trend continues. Eventually, and it is not clear if we are ready yet for this debate, society will have to decide just what it wishes from general practitioners and primary health care teams. If it wishes 24 hour access to medical and nursing advice, whatever the condition, then it must be prepared to fund 24 hour surgeries on a shift system, much as hospitals provide cover. If, however, society values the continuity of care and rich inter-personal relationships that a caring general practice can offer, then it would demand that the night service is reserved for real emergencies and that primary care is respected.

The other side of this debate concerns the services that society believes should be available.

Not only would this assist practices in understanding just what is expected of them, but it will increase accountability. The more we ask to define society's responsibilities, the more society will define ours. However, at present society seems to want everything, all at once, and to pay sparingly for it. This national consumerism is already devaluing the health service.

CLINICAL

As the costs and effectiveness of health care become more explicit within the health service, options will open up for primary care. There has already been a remarkable shift in the clinical burden from secondary care to primary—in 20 years the care of chronic diseases, palliative care, psychotherapy, health promotion, and prevention have all gravitated to the area of lowest cost. In the process the quality and effectiveness of many of these services has increased. Soon hospitals will cease to require an out-patient visit to place a patient on a surgical waiting list, and follow-up appointments after discharge will become rarities. Patients will become accustomed to attending a consultant once or twice only, with repetitive out-patients visits reserved for the few patients for whom clinical control is most appropriately based in secondary care. The range of investigations and procedures in primary care will increase and referrals will be made according to protocols in which the general practitioners and consultants will agree the pre-referral patient work up. This will reduce time and costs, and reduce unnecessary referrals. Many out-patient consultations already occur in health centres or large surgeries, and, as this trend continues, the traditional image of the hospital as the embodiment of secondary care will be eroded. All these changes will increase the burden of health care in general practice, and there will have to be movement of resources from the secondary to the primary sectors. The creation of the unitary commissioning health authorities may facilitate this movement.

THE PRIMARY HEALTH CARE TEAM

The dramatic expansion of the primary health care team in the past two decades has tested the management capacity of many practices, and there are still some smaller practices which have resisted taking on extra staff out of principle. However, most practices now have practice managers, secretaries, receptionists, and practice nurses. Fundholders are integrating their community nurses into their teams, while others have physiotherapists and counsellors.

The most immediate change will be in practice management. All too often practice managers are managers in name only—in reality they are administrators. The new environment is forcing general practitioners to acknowledge that they cannot continue to operate as small businesses which are their personal fiefdom. They are now medium sized businesses that require high quality management. As the role of practice managers increases, so the general practitioners' involvement in day-to-day management will decrease. This is both inevitable and laudable, but it will call into question the assumption that the centre of the practice is a medical partnership. There is no impediment to a practice manager becoming a profit sharing partner in the business (indeed this has happened in the practice of one of the authors). And if it is acceptable to share ownership of the practice with a manager, why not with the nurses and other health professionals?

The clinical core of a primary care team will change, perhaps dramatically, over the next decade. Two complementary trends will drive the change: medical manpower and nursing development. Medical manpower will present a considerable problem. General practitioners will increasingly wish to work less hard, perhaps by having smaller patient lists, and to retire earlier, raising the requirement for numbers of recruits just at a time when recruits are disappearing like melting snow and patient expectations are combining with demography to increase workload. In a discipline based on self-employment and independent contractor status, this is not 'someone else's problem' and will have to be addressed in practices up and down the country. At the same time clinical nurses are freeing themselves of subservience to nurse managers and doctors, both groups having conspired to keep nurses in dependent positions in the health hierarchy. As nurses seek nurse practitioner skills and prise the prescription pad away from the tight grasp of the medical profession, they will increasingly contribute to the clinical endeavour of primary care as equal partners, albeit with different expertise.

Many practices will see that the solution to their medical manpower problems will lie in a new relationship between doctors and nurses, involving a redefinition of roles within a primary health care team. Just as real practice managers will redefine management, so real nurses will redefine clinical care. Patients will come to respect each member of the team for their contribution to primary care and will learn how to seek access to the people who can offer the best solutions to their problems. For doctors, this will represent a new set of personal constructs. No longer the 'owner' and 'leader' of a practice, but increasingly a contributor to a team approach to patient care. The historical pre-eminence of doctors will not disappear overnight, but the evolutionary process will occur incrementally as individual practices find new solutions to their manpower problems.

One 'test case' in which a solution needs to be found is out-of-hours care. The rhetoric of team care sounds bold and fine in the day, but come the evening the team goes home and the telephone is put through to the doctor (at least in practices not using the deputizing service!). The ways in which out of hours medical services are delivered will change, with more options becoming available. Within a few years it will not be expected that a general practice will offer

24 hour care unless it positively chooses to with, certainly, the midnight to six in the morning zone being covered by a local or national alternative. The possibilities include emergency stations, deputizing services, cooperatives, telephone advice services, and nurse visiting. While it is not clear yet which option will predominate, the current option is clearly not going to be acceptable for long.

Looking beyond the preoccupations of doctors and nurses, the primary care team will become more varied. Chiropodists and osteopaths will join us, as will acupuncturists, physical instructors, and group therapists. Our links with social services and occupational therapy will strengthen and community psychiatric nurses will work as closely with us as they do with psychiatrists. These expanding teams will be much more difficult to manage, and it will be impossible for everybody to relate to everybody else. This will lead to various semi-autonomous groupings within the practice which have clear task responsibilities. Only a high quality practice manager will be able to cope in such a world.

TEACHING, TRAINING, AND QUALITY

Throughout the United Kingdom, medical schools are moving their curricula into the community. In the medium term, it is likely that all medical students will be attached throughout their course to a practice and there they will acquire, through a modified apprenticeship, their clinical and behavioural skills. They will attend the medical school for formal didactic teaching (which will be minimal) and they will follow patients through secondary care. At intervals they will undertake an attachment with a hospital firm to gain specific knowledge or skills.

This model of a community based medical school will test the ability and commitment of general practice to teaching, but will offer the best chance of a high quality medical education. Naturally, such a change will have to be accompanied by adequate funding but, unlike the current teaching, it will also operate in a competitive market. Practices that do not offer high quality teaching will be replaced by others that will.

It is commonly believed that vocational training schemes are now so institutionalized that they are immortal. Recent experience in other countries suggests otherwise. New Zealand, for example, has recently reduced funding for vocational training on the basis that professionals should pay for their own education. While such a scenario is unlikely in Britain, not least because the health service has accepted for fifty years that medical education is part of its remit, the future security of vocational training and vocational training schemes depend on the continued demonstration of quality. This will be measured locally in the regular Joint Committee visits to schemes, and nationally in the perceived quality of new entrants.

Postgraduate Deans have taken over the entire budget for hospital training, including posts filled by general practice trainees. This budget initially amounts to half of the salary of junior doctors, and may, in time, include all of it. There are those who wish to see the vocational training budget moved to the postgraduate departments to be managed by Regional Advisers. This would increase the capacity of the general practice educational structure to monitor and regulate postgraduate educational standards.

Certification is a necessity for both the wider profession and the more limited interests of medical educators. An entrance examination for general practice, with minimum standards, is being introduced. At first there are two routes—the MRCGP plus local evidence, and certification by Regional Advisers. In time it is likely that one route will prevail and that it will be the MRCGP which continues to attract more candidates every year. When we can define our educational pathway (compulsory vocational training since 1979), formative assessment of both the educators and the educated, and effective summative assessment to demonstrate that minimum (not minimal) standards are achieved, we will be able to command the confidence of the public.

Once all entrants into our discipline are certificated, and all practices are accredited—note that the term certification is used for individuals and accreditation for organizations—we then need to address the necessity to demonstrate continuing standards. Already re-certification is climbing up the political agenda, and soon practical proposals will be developed. While it will initially be based on a points system for educational attendance, it will soon develop into a more muscular animal. By the end of this decade it is probable that every practice will be involved in a programme of regular visits, say every five years, which will re-accredit it for quality payments, and every general practitioner will be re-certificated as suitable to continue in practice.

Medical audit has, initially, been supported in a ring-fenced world of confidentiality. It will, of course, continue to be the case that individuals and groups will examine emotive and personal areas of care in depth for their own purposes. However, clinical audits will be required in re-accreditation and in re-certification; they will be a normal facet of health needs assessment and will be used to justify resource bids. Just as fundholders are putting quality standards into contracts with provider units, and requiring clinical audits to demonstrate that the standards are met, so those purchasing primary care—mainly the commissioning authorities—will seek to place quality standards on us. Medical audit will, therefore, change into a more amorphous entity with less protection and more openness.

CONTRACT

There seems little likelihood of a return to the pre-reform contract with its absence of expectations on the contractor. Indeed, the purchasers of primary care are going to demand more explicit measures of what they are buying. And they are going to want their contracts to be with practice teams, not individual practitioners. It seems likely that this will be resisted by the profession because of financial insecurity. At first, this will lead to a definition of the range of services available to patients, but soon primary care contracts will cover availability and accessibility, quality of care, and patient education. These are all items, after all, that fundholders impose, as purchasers, on secondary care. The inevitable end point of this trend alongside others already evident—such as locally determined pay for nurses—is a local contract for general practice.

Local contracts will be based on a core national contract which will continue to be negotiated by our national representative body for such matters, the General Medical Services Committee of the BMA. However, areas of local discretion will be significant and will increase. One commissioning authority may decide that cervical cytology is no longer a problem, but teenage pregnancies are a major concern. They may move incentives from one to the other, rewarding practices which can demonstrate a full, accessible service for teenagers.

One by-product of this move will be that the purchasers of primary care—the new commissioning health authorities—will start to price separately each service that we offer and will choose between traditional providers (us) and alternative providers such as private companies. A clearer market place will emerge for all non-core services, especially family planning, obstetrics, minor surgery, and paediatric surveillance. If the profession decides to opt out of its 24 hour responsibility, it will have signalled that all our traditional functions are up for discussion, and there are many who see commercial opportunities in picking off specific tasks. This is precisely the change that solicitors experienced when their hold on conveyancing was loosened.

Another result of these moves will be the definition of minimum contractual standards. We shall see doctors and practices being given notice of discontinuation of their contract with the health service. Thus, general practitioners unable or unwilling to offer an adequate service will no longer be able to operate as independent contractors and will only see patients in primary care under supervision. This vision may sound apocalyptic, but general practice as a whole may benefit if the practices and practitioners offering an unacceptably low standard of care are brought up to acceptable standards. Our Achilles heel has always been the extreme variability of quality of care offered by colleagues, with some embarrassing all of us. If we can encourage the introduction of standards that are credible and relevant then we will all benefit, but that would require our active cooperation. The alternative is that we refuse to contemplate this possibility and the standards are imposed by those who do not understand general practice.

As for the internal market, it is difficult to offer coherent predictions. However, some trends might be discernible. Concern about transaction costs (see Chapter 2) is not just a minor argument about semantics. If fundholding costs more to administer than other forms of purchasing, then there must be clear gains to compensate. A change in political climate might well lead to a reappraisal of the perceived gains with a consequent re-evaluation of fundholding. If this is correct, the future of fundholding is already cast, and it is not positive.

The health service abhors a vacuum and fundholding will not simply disappear. It will change into a general practitioner commissioning process in which practices behave more like health authorities in deploying their funds—in other words money will not be linked to individual patients but to patterns of care—and will be expected to do so under the same constraints and imperatives. Practices will influence secondary care by making strategic purchasing decisions —commissioning—but will have to act within the responsibilities and account-abilities of national programmes such as the Health of the Nation, local priorities, and evidence of health gain. Such a world will seem rather drab to the entrepreneurs of primary care today!

This is, however, one way on which the 'primary care led NHS' can be turned into a reality. By making general practices behave, collectively, like a commissioning authority, with access to public health and health economics advice, the role of the current commissioning authorities will diminish. As total purchasing involves us in every aspect of the health service, and as we demonstrate that we can commission with lower transaction costs (for example management costs) in a way that achieves greater quality with enhanced responsiveness to patient needs, we could become the pivot of the health service. If fundholding falls, all is not lost.

RESEARCH AND ACADEMIA

There is a pronounced move towards support for academic general practice and particularly for the funding of health services research—research into the delivery of care. These trends are likely to continue as long as the health service recognizes that, as a big employer, it devotes too little of its overall budget to research and development, and too little research and development happens where the great majority of care is delivered.

The requirement for academically trained primary care workers will increase and there will be a trend towards non-doctors taking up the challenge. It may be that a new feature will be the academic practice manager, but certainly academic nurses will become more common in primary care. Already the college and regional offices are encouraging the notion of research practices where protected time for research is paid for. The protected time can be allocated to doctors, nurses, other therapists, managers, or administrators. Such practices are unlikely to be effective without extensive support and so regional and national networks are burgeoning. In the north east and on the south coast active networks are encouraging practices to research; national networks, such as the MRC GP Framework or the Weekly Returns Service network, continue to offer opportunities.

In the 1980s, there was a vision of primary care becoming the information supplier to the health service and the pharmaceutical industry. The 'no-cost' option for computers in practices was devised on the assumption that there would be commercial and academic researchers willing to pay for the data. That this proved not to be the case was more a result of inflated expectations of the quality of the data than a failure of the original vision. In the next few years, practices with high quality data on their computer systems will become involved in local and national schemes which will facilitate the aggregation of data and the derivation of information.

As primary care begins to supply the health service's data, the public health physicians can turn away from a concentration on mortality statistics towards the use of incidence, prevalence, and risk behaviour statistics; we can monitor primary care activity; and standards of care data can be used to inform guidelines which are based on the real care of patients in the real world of primary care. The data sharing networks will be ideal for researchers to do hypothesis generation and some hypothesis testing, but routinely collected data imposes severe restrictions on research questions.

In time, general practitioners will chose whether to be undergraduate teachers, vocational trainers, or postgraduate leaders; whether to be involved in data sharing, data gathering for research networks, or researchers in their own right; and whether to contribute as vociferous spectators or active participants in the movement of general practice towards its rightful place as the premier academic discipline in the British health service.

POLITICAL

As primary care increasingly becomes the true centre of the health service, so, paradoxically, will the political power of general practitioners wane. Primary care is so much bigger than general practice, and the Department of Health is recognizing this reality. It is likely, therefore, that consumerism and standard setting will become a predominant influence on the general practice contract and that the widening of the primary health care team will dilute the local influence and power of general practitioners. This trend is already discernible and will accelerate. If the political influence of general practitioners is reduced through the traditional routes, it is likely to increase in the more informal, advisory channels. Every health authority will require expert general practitioner advice, including the Department of Health itself.

CONCLUSIONS

Overall the future looks positive. There are risks, certainly, not least that primary care disappoints the political expectations being vested in it, and the pendulum swings back towards secondary care. The risks seem, on balance, to be smaller than the strengths, and the possibilities for developing primary care seem comparable to those in 1966 when the General Practice Charter was introduced—but from a higher platform. If primary care is to exploit its potential it needs to enhance its teamwork, embrace quality standards, and to augment its educational, academic, and political bases. That should be a sufficient agenda for the next five years!

REFERENCES

1. Royal College of General Practitioners Working Party. *The future general practitioner*: *learning and teaching*. London: BMA, 1972.
2. Royal College of General Practitioners Working Party (Chair: Professor Nigel Stott). *The nature of general medical practice*. London: RCGP, 1995.
3. Jones, R. and Kinmonth, A.-L. (eds.). Evidence based medicine. Oxford: Oxford University Press, 1995.
4. Ridsdale, L. *Evidence-based general practice*. London: Saunders, 1995.
5. Sweeney, K., Gray, D. P., Steele, R., and Evans, P. Use of warfarin in non-rheumatic atrial fibrillation: a commentary from general practice. *British Journal of General Practice* 1995; **45**: 153–8.

Part 2

Problems and solutions

Part 2

Problems and solutions

7 Entering general practice

Preparing to become a principal in general practice is a continuing process throughout vocational training. Young doctors spend three or more years acquiring the necessary clinical and managerial skills to practice independently. They also develop values that will influence their early years as a principal. Evidence of the effectiveness of that training should be collected too. The essential certificate is that from the Joint Committee on Postgraduate Training for General Practice (JCPTGP). This committee is the statutory independent body regulating training for general practice. It is responsible for issuing the certificate of satisfactory completion of vocational training.

Each trainee should ensure that they receive a VTR2 from each of their hospital posts, the form should be signed by the consultant for whom the doctor has worked. Guidance about the suitability of hospital posts may be sought from the JCPTGP or from the Regional Adviser in General Practice. Each trainee should also ensure that they receive a VTR1 form that should be signed by their trainer. Both forms are available from the Regional Adviser's office. VTR forms should be submitted to the Regional Adviser in General Practice who countersigns them and forwards them to the JCPTGP. The forms may be submitted one month before completion of training for general practice or after training has been completed. On receipt of the appropriate forms the JCPTGP issues a certificate of satisfactory completion of training for general practice, without which it is not possible to enter general practice as a principal. Delay can be incurred if training has been undertaken in more than one region as each VTR form has to be countersigned by the Regional Adviser from the region in which the post was held. It is not possible for a trainee to take up work, as a principal, locum, or assistant in general practice without the necessary paperwork:

Philip has been offered a partnership that started within a week of his completion of his training year. He had forgotten to get his VTR2 certificates signed and had to spend time finding the consultants for whom he had worked to obtain their signatures. The delay meant that he was unable to produce his JCPTGP certificate in time for the start of the post, threatening loss of income.

Most trainees aspire to become members of the Royal College of General Practitioners. Entry to the College is now almost exclusively by examination. The exam is not currently mandatory to become a principal, but it is an important assessment of competence in general practice. About 80 per cent of doctors completing vocational training for general practice pass the MRCGP exam.

After 1 September 1996 every doctor completing training for general practice will need to submit themselves to a national assessment, details of the assessment can be obtained from the Regional Adviser in General Practice. It will be possible to gain exemption from certain aspects of this assessment through successfully sitting the MRCGP examination.

As well as the certificate from the Joint Committee that allows a doctor to provide general medical services as a principal in general practice, new principals will need to demonstrate that they are competent in obstetric care, child health surveillance, and minor surgery. Some Family Health Service Authorities (FHSAs) require evidence of competence in these areas, others accept the MRCGP certificate. Inclusion on the child health surveillance, obstetric, and minor surgery lists allows a doctor to be paid to practise his or her skills in these areas, which is part of practising family medicine and brings additional income to the practice.

Child health surveillance

There are national guidelines on the recommended training for child health surveillance; these are obtainable from the Royal College of General Practitioners or from the Regional Adviser in General Practice. Local FHSAs are entitled to set their own standards but most adhere to the national guidelines. Information should be sought from the individual FHSA. A certificate of competence in performance of child health surveillance is required before a candidate can enter the MRCGP examination. This certificate may be acceptable to the FHSA.

Obstetrics

Inclusion on the obstetric list is usually achieved by completing a senior house officer post in obstetrics and/or gynaecology. It is possible to enter the register through an attachment to an obstetric unit during which time the doctor will need to attend antenatal clinics, normal, and abnormal deliveries.[1]

Minor surgery

Many FHSAs allow a basic surgical qualification as the minimum competence in surgical skills, others expect experience after full registration. Other criteria relating to the practice such as the availability of sterilization equipment are usual.

Family planning

Although family planning is an essential part of general practice it is not necessary to have a certificate to undertake the provision of contraceptive services.

CHOOSING A PRACTICE

Finding a practice which matches expectations may be difficult. Many young principals find the early years in practice traumatic, sometimes because they are frustrated at not having the skills to manage change in their practice, but more often because they find the prospect of the change overwhelming. It is a useful exercise to consider carefully what sort of practice you want to work in. It is possible that your needs soon after completing training will be different from those later in life.

John knew that eventually he wanted to work in a single-handed or small practice providing personal care. He also recognized that he wanted to develop his skills in research and teaching. He applied for a lecturer post in the University Department of General Practice, realizing that this was to be for a limited duration.

At this stage it is advisable not be be constrained too much by practical issues but really dream about the future. Writing down a description of your dream will be useful, as the next stage is to think through the practicalities. It may be that your dream practice is incompatible with your spouse's occupation or your domestic situation and compromises will need to be made. Having clarified your own thoughts about the sort of practice that you are seeking, it is likely that you will need to discuss them with your spouse if you have one, or other family members. Finally, it is a good idea to write down the essential characteristics of the practice you are seeking, those which you would like to be present but which are not essential, and those which are definitely negative.

Most practice vacancies are advertised in the journals. Some partnerships, however, still work through word of mouth and some seek the assistance of the Course Organizer or Regional Adviser in General Practice. Many young doctors spend a few months after the completion of vocational training working as a locum. This offers the opportunity of working in different practices that may clarify ideas about the choice of practice. It also allows a young doctor to experience different ways of running a practice which will be useful once established as a partner.

PREPARING AN APPLICATION

Having identified a likely practice, by word of mouth or through an advertisement, you now need to prepare an application. It is usual to submit a typed curriculum vitae with an accompanying hand written letter. Ideally each application should have a new curriculum vitae that should respond to the practice's needs. This may not be practical when a doctor is applying to several posts but each application should have a good quality (not a carbon and preferably not a photocopy) curriculum vitae. There should definitely not be hand written alterations. Ask your trainer or someone whom you respect to look through your

Some aspects of practices to consider before application

Type
  Rural
  Urban
  Dispensing
  Teaching
  Training
Partners
  Age
  Sex
  Values e.g.: Staff development
              Continuing medical education
              Outside activities
              Response to change
Location
  Schools
  Public transport
  Proximity to work for spouse
  Social mix of patients
  Proximity to work for patients
  New building
  New industry
  Proximity to a Vocational Training Scheme
  Proximity to a Medical School
  Proximity to a Postgraduate medical or other education centre
Premises
  Rented
  Practice owned
  Health Authority
Practice team
  Good teamworking
  Involvement of the team in decision making
Patient care
  Single list
  Shared list
  Clinical/audit meetings
  Clinical management protocols
Practice income
  High earning
  Outside practice income
Out of hours
  Availability of deputizing service/co-operative
  Practice rota within the practice or including others
Record systems
  Lloyd George
  A4
  Computer
Fundholding
  Currently fundholding
  Preparing to fundhold
  Against fundholding
Local GP population
  Active continuing medical education
  Active on purchasing consortium
Local hospital
  Good working relationships
  Access to investigations
Local support services
  Health visiting
  District nursing
  Social services
  Other support services

Areas to be included in a curriculum vitae

Name
Date of birth
Address, with day and evening telephone numbers
Marital status
Nationality
General education
Medical school
Qualifications
Date of full registration with GMC
Prizes and awards
Previous appointments
Present appointments
Career plans
Special skills
Publications
Teaching experience
Interests outside work
Referees

---

curriculum vitae, ask them to be critical. Does it present you in your best light? Is it clear what qualities you would be bringing to a partnership?

If a photograph is asked for, make sure that it is included. It is wise to let referees know about your applications and include their telephone number in the application. General practice is still a small community and a referee may know one of the prospective partners.

If there is time, it would be sensible to visit the practice area. If it is unfamiliar, is it what you expected? When you are short-listed, if you are serious about the job, you must visit the practice, arranging a time with the practice manager or one of the partners. Seek information before you go, your Trainer or Course Organizer may be familiar with the practice and be aware of its strengths and areas for concern.

It is a good idea to refer to the short-list of qualities that you were seeking. How does the practice match up? There is obviously a balance between finding out enough information for you to make a decision and appearing critical. Most general practitioners are proud of their practice and most think that they do a good job. Phrase your questions carefully and be aware of sensitive areas. The 'informal' visit should be used wisely. Many practices interview in the evenings or weekends, this may be the only opportunity to observe the practice in action. Try to meet other members of the health care team especially those who are attached to the practice and may have less loyalty. Use the time with the practice manager or one of the partners to test the ground for the interview, what sort of partner are they looking for? Be prepared to be assessed yourself. Some partnerships like to observe a potential partner consulting, others may be looking for particular characteristics and may ask you to complete a personality questionaire such as 'Belbin'.[2]

THE INTERVIEW

The interview may take a variety of forms, be prepared for anything from a formal panel with a professional interviewer to an informal gathering over a meal. Some partnerships like to meet the spouses of potential partners before making a final decision, others may wait until an appointment has been made. It would be advisable to find out the format of the interview on the informal visit. The interview will also be an important opportunity for you to observe the partnership. Be ready with some questions that will help you decide if you can work with these doctors.

Probably the most important aspect of choosing a practice is the partners. Do you feel you could work with them? Do you share their values on patient care? What are their thoughts on fundholding and are they the same as your own? How are practice decisions taken? Why is the outgoing partner leaving? Does it feel a happy partnership? What part do the spouses play? Will that match with your own spouse's expectations?

Finally, there are the terms and conditions of service to consider. These questions may be best left to a second interview. Start with a question that is unlikely to cause offence such as 'What is the weekly timetable?' Judge carefully how it is received and whether you should proceed on this occasion. Listen carefully to the answers you receive and be ready with subsidiary questions without appearing aggressive. Asking questions about the partnership can be difficult. It is essential that you understand the commitment and the rewards of the partnership but asking delicate questions can be hard. There is always the fear that you may give the impression of laziness or greed. The skills involved are very similar to those you learned in eliciting information from patients. A pleasant, quiet tone of voice, asking open questions without embarrassment is usually the most successful method. Your Trainer, Course Organiser, or a friend might be willing to role play this part of the interview with you, using a video-recorder so that you can try out different ways of asking the questions.

MAKING A DECISION

It is unlikely that any one practice will have all the qualities that you listed at the initial exercise and you may have to reach a compromise. It may be that the practice has many of the features that you are looking for but that there would need to be some changes to achieve all of them. How easy do you think it would be to implement these changes? How easily could you work in the practice

---

Some questions to consider for interview

How are decisions taken in the practice?

How often do the partners meet?
>   Formally
>   Informally

What plans does the partnership have for the future?

How are decisions about on call rota and holiday taken?

What role does the practice manager take in the practice?

What are the relationships like with the primary health care team?

What are the relationships like with other agencies?
>   FHSA
>   Local hospitals

How are repeat prescriptions handled?

What is the policy on telephone prescribing?

What is the policy on out-of-hours cover?

What is the practice involvement in maternity care, child health screening, clinical, and managerial audit?

How are rooms used in the practice, will the incoming partner have their own room?

How does the practice assess the quality of the service it is providing?

What audits are ongoing, what have been the findings in the previous twelve months?

---

before the changes were made? Are there any other factors, such as another partner likely to leave or a partner wanting to move in the same direction as yourself, that would assist the change?

APPLICATION FOR A SINGLE-HANDED VACANCY

Applying for a single-handed vacancy has many aspects in common with an application for a partnership. Many of the preliminary stages are likely to be the same; however, there are aspects that differ. Applications for a single-handed partnership are made to the FHSA. It is usual to complete a series of forms which are submitted to the FHSA. The forms will ask candidates to set out their expected surgery hours and the times of additional clinics. The appointments

---

**Some questions relating to the terms and conditions of the
partnership to think about**

What will be the likely weekly timetable?
Make sure you are aware of the other partners' timetables as well as your
    own. Is there an even distribution of workload? Is the workload of the
    practice audited?

What will the on call rota be?
Is this sharing with another practice? You may be told that you are
    working one night a week and one weekend in four when you enter a
    four-partner practice, but if this is combined with a neighbouring
    practice and only the four junior partners do the on call, will you be
    happy? What happens at holiday time? Will the night on call be fixed,
    that is, every Friday?

What is the intended profit share?

What are the arrangements for working to parity?
Will there be mutual assessment? If so, on what grounds?

Will the new partner take on the list of the outgoing partner?
If not, at what stage will the new partner be expected to take on patients?

What arrangements does the practice have for splitting external income?

What are the arrangements for taking annual leave and study leave?
Will you be able to take school holidays or will you take last place in the
    queue? Will your study leave be cancelled if the senior partner wants
    to take a holiday?

---

committee is likely to be made up of representatives from the FHSA and local
general practitioners. Most appointments committees will be trying to identify a
doctor who will be looking to the future; as well as seeking someone who will
provide the best care for the practice population, they will be looking for a
doctor who will contribute to the general practice community. A recent publication suggests that the MRCGP should be the usual standard for appointment to
a single-handed vacancy.[3]

If it is possible, find out about the practice and the population it serves. Are
there special features that need care over surgery times such as a local factory
or market day? Is there potential for innovation such as the introduction of a
child health surveillance clinic? What do the local population want from their
general practitioner? What changes will you anticipate? A short and long-term
business plan with likely costings will impress the selection committee. What
about adjacent practices? Are they applying for the list? Is there potential for an

on-call rota? At the interview be prepared to answer questions about your likely budget requirements, in particular changes in staff, introduction of computers, or changes to the building. Be prepared to justify the expenditure.

George was applying for a single-handed vacancy. He spent time looking round the practice area and at the practice premises. He could see that without major changes to the record systems and the introduction of practice computers he would find difficulty working in the practice. He set about writing a clear plan for achievement of change, including the likely staff requirements that he submitted with his application. He was successful.

THE PRACTICE AGREEMENT

No matter how well you seem to get on with your partners, a practice agreement or contract is essential. Hopefully, having signed it, the agreement will be put away and never referred to again. However, without an agreement it may be difficult to defend your position if things go wrong.

Jane entered partnership soon after completing training. After six months mutual assessment she was offered a permanent partnership. She and the partners agreed the profit sharing ratios as she worked to parity and agreed that she would gradually build up her list, taking on new registrations from a new estate that was being built. Three months later, Jane discovered she was pregnant; although it was earlier than she and her boyfriend had intended they were both thrilled. Jane told the partners her good news at the next meeting. She was totally taken aback when two days later the practice manager handed her a letter asking her to leave the partnership. Without a practice agreement and without her own list Jane had very little option.

Discussion: There are two things that give general practitioners security, one is the partnership agreement, the other is having a list of patients. The partnership agreement is very important and should contain basic elements. When a general practitioner has a list of patients they are entitled to take their list if the partnership splits. In the early stages of a doctor's career it is likely that many patients will stay with the familiar practice but over time they will build a relationship with the new doctor and may prefer to move. Most partnerships do not give an incoming partner a list until they have passed the assessment period. This avoids unnecessary risk and is quite reasonable. Some partnerships continue to refuse to allow a junior partner to sign on patients, or maintain very uneven lists. If this is so there is cause for concern. Jane had passed the assessment period and if she had replaced an outgoing partner she should have expected to take on a list.

The British Medical Association produces a model practice agreement. As a minimum, a practice agreement should contain statements about maternity leave, sick leave, distribution of profits, the contribution of non-NHS earnings to the partnership, management of practice staff, partnership decisions, partnership taxation, study leave, and holiday entitlement. Advice from a solicitor is important when drawing up a practice agreement, although the more technical legal language may be best avoided. At this stage it is advisable to clarify whether any financial contribution to the practice equipment or building is needed.

INVESTING IN A PRACTICE

A doctor at the beginning of their career may worry about investing in a practice. Taking on one mortgage may seem bad enough but the prospect of taking on two may seem impossible. Before rejecting the idea of investing in practice premises seek some advice from your trainer and other local general practitioners. The short-term hardships are often more than outweighed by the long-term investment. Before young doctors commit themselves to investment in a building they should have a valuation of the property to be clear that they are contributing an appropriate sum of money and that they will receive a corresponding benefit from any notional rent. It is quite permissable for the partnership share of the building to be different from that of the profit share. Advice from an accountant familiar with general practice finance would be useful. Even if an incoming partner is not expected to invest in the building it is likely that there will be a need to invest in fixtures and fittings, computer equipment, and pharmaceutical stock. These items are often referred to as fixed capital. It would be usual for the property and fixed capital to be assessed by the partnership when a partner retires or leaves the practice, there will then be an arrangement made for the incoming partner to contribute.

PRACTICE ACCOUNTS

Before entering a partnership it is important to study the practice accounts. It may be helpful to seek professional advice to interpret the accounts. It is important to observe trends in income and expenditure, and in particular to consider the overall profits and how they are made up. Is a large share of the practice income derived from the outgoing partner's non-NHS activity? Most practices would expect an incoming partner to ask to see the accounts. Any difficulty must be viewed with concern.

GETTING STARTED

As the big day to start in the new partnership approaches there are still fine details that need attention. There are forms that need to be submitted to the FHSA: Joint Committee Certificate, Child Health Surveillance, Minor Surgery, Obstetric Register, specimen signatures for prescriptions and, if there is more than twelve months gap between completing vocational training and starting as a principal, certificates of attendance at Postgraduate Education Activities. It is important to clarify the timetable with the practice manager, and perhaps spend some time learning the geography of the practice area, for which a map may be important.

REFERENCES

1. Statement of Fees and Allowances. Leeds: NHS Executive, 1996. (Section 31.19, clause 6).
2. Belbin, M. *Management teams: why they succeed or fail.* London: Butterworth Heinemann, 1991.
3. National Association for Health Authorities and Trusts (NAHAT). *Partners in learning: Developing postgraduate training and continuing medical education for general practice.* London: NAHAT, 1994.

8 Relationships

General practice, like many other professional partnerships, is dependent on good relationships between partners. It is also dependent on good relationships with other people working with, and associated with, the practice. The root of much discontent in general practice often lies in lack of communication or misunderstanding of other people's points of view. Good relationships make life pleasant which reflects on our care of our patients. However, as in many other areas of our lives, time needs to be spent on building relationships and understanding each others' roles in and outside the practice.

THE PARTNERS

In an earlier chapter we considered various ways in which you might assess the beliefs and motivating factors of the partners before joining the practice. Now that you are in the practice you will have opportunity to consider them at leisure. In this chapter there are exercises which may help you reflect on relationships within the partnership. An essential aspect of all organizations is healthy relationships; although it may be possible to manage in the early years in partnership without spending time building relationships and understanding the other partners' views, if there is not mutual respect resentment and difficulties soon build up. Try to get to know your partners socially as well as professionally, observe and listen to them and their families. Your partners and their spouses are likely to have a high investment in the practice, and, although they may be seeking change they may not be ready to have it thrust upon them. It may help relationships if each partner understands the other partner's perceptions of the practice and how they would like it to change. Exercise 8.1 may help you and your partners to understand each other better. It is important to take time to listen to each other and identify ways that may allow each person to benefit. Of course, not all dreams are achievable but compromises may be reached:

Dr Smith was a keen sailor. Every weekend if he were not on call for the practice, he worked on his yacht which was his pride and joy. Dr Smith was in partnership with Dr Jones, who was married to an estate agent. Dr Jones's wife had to work most weekends, but she could take time off during the week. Dr Jones offered to swap some of his midweek commitments for some of Dr Smith's weekend duty. Dr Smith was delighted. They discussed their idea and then brought it to a partnership meeting. The other partners agreed to the swap for a trial period of six months.

Discussion: Both Dr Smith and Dr Jones benefited from the arrangement. Before they set up any changes, they discussed their plans with the partnership.

Exercise 8.2 helps the partners to extend their aspirations for themselves and think about the practice. It is the first part of our strategic planning exercise.

Exercise 8.1   To identify each partners' personal aspirations

Each partner should undertake this exercise individually. Sharing the results will help you to understand each others' perception.

1. Draw two large circles separated by a line. Label the one on the left *The present* and the one on the right *The future*.

2. Divide each circle into segments, like a pie chart. Each segment on the left circle should represent how you *feel* you spend your time now. Each segment of the right circle should represent how you would like to spend your time.

3. It is likely that there will be a difference between the two circles. Take time to think why that is.

4. Now try to think what you need to do to achieve your dream.

5. There are certain factors that will help you achieve your desired time allocation and certain factors that will prevent you from achieving it. Make a list of each:

Factors that will help you in reaching your goal   **Factors that will prevent you from reaching your goal**

These two exercises (8.1 and 8.2) may help you to understand your partners' values more clearly, but may not explain why the partnership behaves as it does. Meredith Belbin studied the working of management teams and has written his observations in an easy to read book.[1] His conclusions are as pertinent to general practice as they are to management teams. He observed teams of people working together and noted that individuals took up certain roles within the team. He noted that when a team was composed of individuals who took different team roles it was more successful than when team members tended to take the same roles. A brief outline of the roles defined by Belbin is included in Table 8.1.

You may have been thinking about your practice team as you read the description and your team may enjoy completing the Belbin self-perception inventory questionnaire.[1] Having considered the eight important team roles, can you identify any roles that are missing from your team? Could they be filled by a team member outside the partnership, perhaps the practice manager? Can you see why conflicts appear in your partnership? We all tend to gravitate to people who are similar to ourselves and choosing a partner is no exception. Many practice partnerships are composed of three or four like-minded people who mix well together but if the team is to be successful some members of the partnership may have to take up a role that fits uncomfortably:

Exercise 8.2   To identify each partners' aspirations for the practice
(From Pendleton & King)

In this exercise ask the partnership to discard any constraints and imagine how they would really like their practice to be.

1. Each partner should imagine that it is five years in the future and that the practice has been given an award for merit in five areas.

2. Each partner should take about thirty minutes to write down the areas that he or she would like to be awarded a merit for excellent performance.

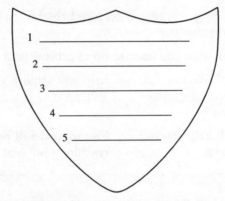

1 _____

2 _____

3 _____

4 _____

5 _____

3. Each partner should take about ten minutes to present his vision of the practice to the other partners. The exercise is helped if each partner can write his five vision statements on a large sheet of paper.

The partners in the Happy Valley practice were fun to work with. They bubbled with ideas and enjoyed evenings out together. Somehow, their ideas never seemed to take shape in the partnership. Some never got further than the lively discussion in the restaurant while others never seemed to work out as they had intended. Soon after the 1990 contract, the senior partner, Dr Jolly, appeared distant. He no longer came to the practice meals or if he did he remained a bit apart. The other partners thought that it was the strain of the new contract, until one day he exploded in the reception area, angry at the lack of support he was getting from the other partners in achieving the expected targets.

Discussion: The partners in the practice enjoyed working together, but their makeup was such that none of them took an obvious leadership role. When leadership was essential, as in implementing the new contract, the task fell to the senior partner who liked the mantle no more than the others.

Exercises 8.1 and 8.2 may have helped you understand your partners a little better. It would be quite reasonable for a brand new partner not to rush into inviting the other partners to reflect on the practice direction and what they

Table 8.1 Belbin personality types

Personality type	Description of personality
Team leaders	
Shaper	These individuals tend to be highly strung, outgoing, and dynamic. They drive forward, always trying to complete the task and move to the next one. They are prone to irritation and impatience.
Chairman	These people tend to be self-confident and in control. They welcome contributors without prejudice and have a clear sense of objectives. They may lack intellect and creative ability.
Ideas people	
Plant	Plants tend to be individualistic, serious minded, and unorthodox. They have a capacity for imagination and knowledge. They tend to disregard practical details and protocol.
Resource investigators	These people tend to be extrovert, enthusiastic, curious, and communicative. They enjoy contacting others and exploring new ideas, translating them into their own working environment. They are liable to lose interest once the initial fascination has passed.
People who work for the team	
Team worker	These individuals tend to be socially orientated, sensitive, and interested in people and communication. They possess an ability to respond to people and situations and promote the team spirit. They may be indecisive in a crisis.
Company worker	These individuals are conservative and dutiful. They tend to have excellent organizing ability, they are practical and hardworking. They may lack flexibility and be unresponsive to unproven ideas.
Evaluators and completers	
Monitor evaluator	Monitor evaluators are likely to be sober, unemotional, and prudent. They have an inbuilt immunity from enthusiasm but are excellent at making shrewd judgements. They may lack inspiration and be unable to motivate others easily.
Completer-finisher	Completer-finishers are often painstaking, orderly, and conscientious, they have a capacity to follow-through and aim for perfection. They tend to worry about detail and may be reluctant to 'let go'.

were contributing to it. If you have taken time to think about your own strengths and weaknesses and your intended direction for yourself and your practice, it will help you to contribute more positively in the partnership.

One area where it is important for all the partners to work together is care of the patients, particularly where the practice runs a shared list. Most doctors are enthusiastic about discussing clinical issues, usually early morning or coffee time will find groups of doctors and other health professionals discussing patients. The partnership may be less enthusiastic about organized, formal clinical meetings and setting protocols for disease management. The new partner may be viewed as someone who is bringing the latest ideas or someone who threatens to expose clinical ignorance. Take time to reflect on your partners. How do you think each of them view your contribution to the practice? What has made you reach those conclusions? What might you do about it?

SPOUSES

In Chapter 11 on the health of doctors we discuss life events and their effect on our health. Throughout this book we have focused on principals in their practices; many young doctors will have a life-partner who is surviving similar traumas. The term spouse is used to differentiate between partners in the practice; marriage is not essential to reading this section. About 70 per cent of young principals will have a spouse who is working outside the home. Many are married to other doctors, some of whom will be general practitioners. During the early years, the practice seems to consume all the working day, and if there is urgency to complete tasks, most of the evening as well. Our families start to become irritated when we bring work home; our partners become irritated if we leave work undone. Having settled into your practice it may be time to consider your spouse and how they see the future. As with other relationships it is important to set time aside, and you may both need time to think individually, Exercise 8.1 could equally be used with your spouse. When a general practitioner and their family live in the community in which they practise, there are obvious advantages in terms of travelling and understanding the community. However, it may pose considerable stress on our families if they feel that they are constantly being judged. Listen to your family, how does your work affect them?

The aspect of our lives that we feel impinges on our family life the most is 'on call'. Although the green grass of our consultant friends may appear more attractive, the changes in the Health Service are signalling that on call for hospital consultants may be as busy as ours. The national survey of all general practitioners in 1992 indicated that on call was a burden to most of us. Alternatives are currently being proposed but it is likely that we will be faced with on call responsibility for a while yet. Ways of coping are considered in Chapter 11. Our spouses find on call equally stressful. Their anxiety may be alleviated by a mobile telephone, knowing that you can be contacted quickly may reduce their fear of coping in an emergency, and it may also allow them the freedom to leave the house.

THE PATIENTS

One of the strengths of British general practice is the system of the registered list. The registered list gives patients access to a personal doctor who is familiar with their medical and social history. Starting in practice is probably the most difficult time, when we are unfamiliar with our patients and they are not clear about our capabilities and our way of working. Even when we take over a list we still have to build our relationship with our patients. It is often not until a general practitioner changes practice that the importance of 'reputation' becomes clear.

It can be difficult when we dislike a patient, but it is important that we are aware of our feelings and try to prevent them from interfering with our care. Sometimes it helps to try to disentangle why we feel as we do about patients. The term 'heartsink patients' has recently been used to describe patients who dampen our spirits when they walk through the door. Many have chronic illnesses that both doctor and patient have difficulty coping with, others may have little serious disease but may have undergone an unexpectedly high number of investigations. It is difficult in a single year for registrars to grasp fully the impact of heartsink patients. Many young principals' groups find this a useful topic for discussion.

It can be equally difficult when our patients are our friends; it can be difficult to remain objective without appearing detached and uncaring. It can be difficult when members of the same family give conflicting views on emotional problems. There are no easy answers. Balint pioneered work discussing the effect of the doctor on the patient and the patient on the doctor. Some young principals' groups use this style of working, some have found that a clinical psychologist helps to retain reality and clarify thoughts.

THE PRIMARY HEALTH CARE TEAM

Many of the difficulties of young principals have focused on relationships with the partners in the practice. As primary care moves from a doctor based discipline to one that involves the whole primary care team, we need to consider our relationships with the members of our team. Stott has helped our thinking in relation to the core team and the extended team.[2] However, each practice will work slightly differently, and it is important to work effectively in your own practice. Exercise 8.3 may help you to think about your team.

In Chapter 9, on managing change, we consider motivation. The doctor often remains an important motivator of the primary health care team. Your team, especially the employed staff, will look to you for leadership and will be inspired by your enthusiasm. It is likely that you have already been inspired by a colleague or friend with whom you have worked; it may be useful to reflect on their leadership qualities that inspired you and consider whether their style would suit your way of working. Sometimes it is inappropriate for the doctor to be the leader of the team. In the care of the disabled, the community nurse is likely to know more about the patient and the services available. Take time to reflect how you have felt when you have not been allowed to contribute fully in

> **Exercise 8.3**   To reflect on the members of the primary health care team
>
> Take time to ask yourself these questions. Writing down answers helps to focus your thoughts.
>
> 1. Who do I consider to be in my primary health care team?
> 2. What are each of the individual members' strengths?
> 3. When we meet in a group do we take time to listen to each other?
> 4. How would I feel if a member of the team made a justified critical comment about my work?
> 5. How would I feel about another of the health care team leading on patient care?
> 6. How would I feel about another member of the health care team chairing practice meetings?

a discussion. Do you and your partners sometimes limit other members' contributions to the practice?

YOUNG PRINCIPALS

Young principals' groups have become an important feature of the early years in general practice. They provide support and encouragement that often seems to be lacking in the practice. Away from patients and our staff we feel able to be open about our difficulties. By working together solutions emerge. The group is likely to be an important prop during the early years. Groups need to be nurtured too. There needs to be time for each member of the group to take the floor when they need. The old adage 'God gave us two ears, two eyes, and one mouth for them to be used in that ratio' applies as much to working in groups as it does to many other aspects of general practice.

THE OUTGOING PARTNER

Perhaps the most difficult relationship for a new partner to handle is the one with the outgoing partner. Often there is little opportunity to get to know him, yet most of the working day in the early years is spent in his shadow. Many of our senior colleagues leave their practices after years of service. Most have built the practice from almost nothing, seeing two major changes in general practice and many more changes within the National Health Service. Despite all the difficulties they continued to provide care for their patients and introduced change in the practice to meet the growing needs of the health service. Their systems may not be the same as the training practice's from which the young partner is emerging but the senior partner has always been proud of them. The patients are likely to remember the old doctor fondly; they may not take easily to a new doctor:

Paul took over the list of a retiring seventy years old doctor who had worked in the practice for over forty years. The record systems were haphazard with very sparse entries, there was no appointment system or preventive work. Paul was surprised to find that the patients liked this way of working. They wondered why he needed to keep records, unlike Dr Good who had kept all the information about them and their families in her head.

It can be counterproductive to alter a previous doctor's management or treatment plans too rapidly unless there are urgent clinical indications, as some patients are extremely loyal.[3] There will always be those patients who are looking for a fresh face and are keen to accept new ways of working. Caution needs to be exerted with this group too, since it would be inappropriate to imply that the doctor who has looked after them for the past twenty years was out of date or incompetent. Alternatively, a new partner may be taking over from one of the most able general practitioners in the area and may have a very hard act to follow. If there is an opportunity, spend time with the outgoing partner finding out about him. What sort of general practitioner was he? What does he value about medicine? What can he tell you about the history of the practice? You may learn a lot about the practice as well as learning how to handle the patients.

REFERENCES

1. Belbin, M. *Management teams. Why they succeed or fail.* London: Butterworth Heinemann, 1991.
2. Stott, N. *The nature of general medical practice.* London: RCGP, 1995.
3. Cartwright, A. and Anderson, R. *General practice revisited. A second study of patients and their doctors.* London: Tavistock, 1981.

9 Managing change

At times it seems that the National Health Service has gone through so many changes since the 1990 reforms were introduced that we have all suffered excess. However, there are still plans to move more patient care to primary care and we must be ready to face this challenge. Many practices seem to look to the junior partner to update them on the latest trends. This chapter endeavours to introduce the new principal to procedures that will help them to plan and manage change and respond to imposed change.

WHY CHANGE?

There has been considerable anger among general practitioners to the imposed changes of the 1990 contract, but if we reflect on the progress of general practice since the inception of the National Health Service in 1948 it will become obvious that many more changes were introduced by the general practitioners themselves. Shortly after the introduction of the National Health Service, Joseph Collings was commissioned to review the current state of general practice.[1] He described in detail the poor state of general practice; inadequate practice premises, general practitioners coping with vast list sizes, and the lamentable morale of the doctors because of compromised standards. Fortunately our predecessors were skilled enough to see how general practice might develop and manage the change.

Medical knowledge and technology are continually advancing and it has become obvious in recent years that caring for patients in hospital is often inefficient and not an option preferred by patients. Primary care has to continue to advance in order to provide the level of care expected by society. General practitioners have played an important part in leading many of the changes in the provision of health care; some have anticipated changes, and prepared for them, while a small group seemed to bury their heads until the changes were upon them:

Mark joined a practice on 1 April 1990, the day of the introduction of the new contract. During his first week he asked the practice manager how the practice was comparing with the expected targets on immunization and cervical cytology. He was dismayed to find out that the practice had no systems in place to monitor and achieve the expected targets. James, his colleague from the day release course, started as a principal about the same time. The practice that James joined had been keeping manual records of immunization and cervical cytology for many years and was in the process of transferring the information onto a computer.

Discussion: The two practices contrast the approach to the introduction of the new contract, one convincing themselves that it will never happen and the other preparing for the imposed change.

Before changing a current way of working we need to reflect why we need to change. Reasons for introducing change include:

1. current systems or practices are outdated;

2. dissatisfaction with the current system;

3. a new partner or member of staff bringing new ideas;

4. patient dissatisfaction with the current system;

5. change in contract/statement of fees and allowances;

6. in response to findings of audit.

Sometimes we have little choice. Change is introduced from outside the practice. Some changes have been introduced thoughtfully and with consultation, others have been imposed without consultation and explanation resulting in bitterness and resentment. The 1990 contract for general practice is perhaps one of the most well remembered imposed changes. There is still considerable anger within general practice at the way that this was introduced. However, before we decry the Government, we should check our own processes so that we do not impose change on others without adequate consultation:

The town centre practice was fortunate to have an excellent health visitor attached to the practice. She virtually ran the baby clinic, the patients adored her, and she was able to make sure that they all attended for immunization. One day she told the partners that her managers had informed her that she was to be transferred to a neighbouring new town practice, which had a high incidence of problem families. The partners in the town centre practice were very angry.

Discussion: The practice and the health visitor were understandably annoyed when their current working arrangements were disrupted. Discussion between the nurse manager and the practice could have played to the practice's pride in their achievement and allowed them to propose that their health visitor should be be seconded to the new town practice for a predetermined time.

INTRODUCING CHANGE

It is most unlikely that any young principal will join a practice that is perfect in every way. There will always be modifications and improvements that can be made to management systems and patient care. Introducing change can be extremely difficult in the early years in general practice. There is no one correct way, each practice and each situation will be different. General practice is a very individual occupation; we change practice infrequently and we are less exposed to observation and criticism of our work than many other professions. Before launching into major alterations to the working of the practice, it may be worth taking time to reflect on the history of the practice and which members of the practice have a special affinity to the current systems.

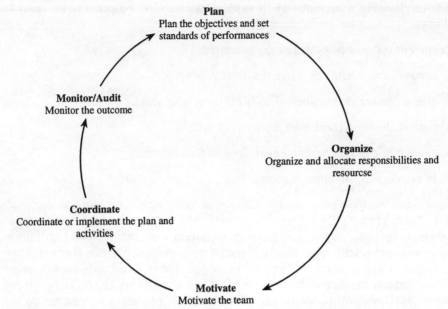

Fig. 9.1. The management cycle. (From Irvine, Huntington. *Management appreciation.* Royal College of General Practitioners.)

Planned change

An increasing number of practices are using strategic planning to identify their likely modifications for the coming year. The partners meet annually to review their previous year's plan and set targets for the coming year. Many use the steps that have been set out in our strategic planning exercise; they share their vision, identify the helping and hindering forces, and identify a plan. Each aspect of the plan should be supplemented by an audit of the current activity and a plan with a time-scale for introducing change. (Fig. 9.1)

Change in response to imposed change

The National Health Service is undergoing considerable modifications and it is likely that general practice will encounter further changes. As these changes are introduced, each practice will need to reconsider its current way of working. A new principal may choose to use the imposed changes as an opportunity to unlock the practice's way of working. Offering to manage the change that the practice will need to make may be met by great relief by the other partners.

Change in response to a serious event in the practice

The practice may suffer a mishap or disaster which makes them reconsider their current way of working. A new principal may use the opportunity to propose that the practice take stock of its current working arrangements and looks at modifications:

Sam was a new partner in the town centre practice. Ever since he had joined the practice he had felt uncomfortable that the practice was too relaxed about reviewing patients whose repeat medication was held on the computer. About six months after he joined the practice, a patient on long-term anti-coagulation therapy was admitted to hospital with a massive gastrointestinal bleed. When the partners gathered to discuss when had happened, Sam used the opportunity to put forward a suggestion that all patients on repeat medication should have a review date. After that review date reception staff should not be authorized to issue a repeat prescription.

Discussion: Sam was aware that the system of repeat prescribing needed review, but he was wary of appearing critical too early. When the opportunity arose he used it to take the practice to where he wanted it to be.

In response to an idea generated by the partners

One or more of the partners or the practice manager may encounter a new system, possibly by visiting another practice or at an educational event. They may feel that the new system is an improvement on current activity and wish to introduce it.

PRINCIPLES IN THE MANAGEMENT OF CHANGE

The fundamental questions in managing change are:

1. Where do we want to be?

2. Where are we now?

3. How are we going to get there?

4. What will we need and what will we need to do to get there?

5. How will we know when we have got there?

6. If we do not get there will we know why?

Where do we want to be?

The first step in making changes is to decide where you want to be. Throughout this part of the book we have referred to setting the vision. It is an important aspect of improving quality in any general practice. Without an idea of where you want to be it will be very difficult to go forward. Many new principals seem to enter general practice with wonderfully clear aspirations, which seem to dull and become overwhelmed with the enormous task of coping with everyday workload. Try to create some time in your working week for thinking about the future, perhaps while you are walking the dog or relaxing in the bath.

Although it is important to have your own clear ideas of where you want to be, if you are working in a partnership those ideas should fit in with your partners. If you are single handed, you may have constraints of finances, building, or staff. Thinking about the whole practice in the future may be too difficult and it may help to break it down into manageable sections. The Royal College of General Practitioners has set out a clear framework for appraising a practice.[2] It defines good practice in terms of:

- availability and accessibility
- communication
- professional values
- clinical competence.

Another document that you might find helpful in setting goals is *Fellowship by Assessment*.[3] Although the idea of Fellowship by Assessment may be daunting and distant, it is achievable and it may be something which you may want to work towards, either implicitly or overtly with the support of your partners.

Once you have established your own ideas about the future of the practice you will need to share them with your partners and practice manager. How this is done will depend on the ethos of the practice. Some partnerships may not be ready for a strategic planning meeting; some may resent time allocated to thinking about the future. Although there may not be formal meetings in which to raise the subject of the future, there will be times when the partners are together, maybe over coffee or reading the post in the morning. General discussion may help you to understand how each of your partners sees the future. All practices have to produce an annual report for the FHSA; many produce an additional internal report for their own purposes. Either of these may be a way of getting the partnership to think about the future. A page in the practice annual report could be used to set practice targets for the coming year and may be the start of forward planning. If your practice is ready for strategic planning it would be useful to refer to the exercise on page 130.

Where are we now?

If a primary health care team is going to manage change effectively, it needs to understand where it is starting from. It may be easy to look at your ideal practice and describe the converse. This may not help you in managing change. Your practice behaves as it does through an imbroglio of personalities and history. Only when you understand the intricacies of both of these will you be able to move forward, certain in the knowledge that the whole of the team is with you. The next stage is to understand what motivates you and the others around you. If you do not present your proposed change in a way that appeals to others it is likely to be doomed. Understanding the motivation of the members of your primary health care team, especially your partners', is important to the success of your project. Spend time with them, listen to them, watch them at work, watch their body language as well as listening to the words they speak.

How are we going to get there?

How the change is managed will depend on the team, the starting point, and the finishing point. It is important to be clear about your ultimate goal; if you are not, you may waver from your path. It is essential to consider the factors that will help you achieve your goal and those that will hinder, and that you weigh up the costs of each route.

Understanding yourself

It may sound banal that the first stage in managing change is to understand yourself, the role you like to take in the team, what motivates you, and your preferred management style. You may like to complete the Belbin Inventory (see Chapter 8) to understand yourself and the role you like to play in your team. There are a few common factors that are likely to motivate you and others in your team:

- knowing that you are doing a job well
- gaining the respect of peers and colleagues
- increased status
- financial rewards.

It is likely that the first two factors on the list are significant in motivating you. They may be important to your staff. Many general practitioners assume that their staff are not interested in improving their performance. They tend to control the work themselves. It may help to complete Exercise 9.1 to understand what motivates you and Exercise 9.2 which should help you understand more about your management style.

Perhaps the most difficult aspect of entering general practice as a new partner is learning how to handle your partners. While reflecting on your management style with your staff, it may be prudent to reflect on your relationships with each of your partners. Exercise 9.3 helps you consider your relationships with your partners. It may seem cumbersome to have taken time to reflect on partnership dynamics; it will, however, always be time well spent. Many young principals' groups spend a great deal of time on this aspect of practice. You may find it helpful to discuss some of these exercises in your young principals' group.

Exercise 9.1   To identify personal motivators and depressors

1. Take time to reflect on what motivates you.

2. Reflect on the aspects of work that you enjoy and the times when you feel despondent.

3. Write two lists, one of the situations which made you feel good and one when you felt despondent.

Exercise 9.2   To consider your management style.
(From Irvine, Huntington. *Management Appreciation.* Royal College of General Practitioners)

Take time to reflect on your style of management, ask yourself the following questions:

1. Do I create a social climate in which subordinates feel respected?

2. Do I treat mistakes as opportunities for learning and growth?

3. Do I help my subordinates discover what they need to learn?

4. Do my staff members have responsibilities for designing and carrying out their own learning experiences?

5. Do my staff members engage in self appraisal and personal planning for performance improvement?

6. Do I permit or encourage innovation and experiments to change the accepted way of doing things, if the plan proposed appears possible?

7. Am I aware of the development issues which concern my staff?

8. Do I try to implement a problem finding and problem solving strategy to involve my staff in dealing with day to day problems and longer range issues?

Moving forwards

Now that you are clear where you want to be and where you and the practice are coming from, it is time to think about how to get there. Many of us make the grave mistake of trying to achieve too much too quickly. Change takes time and

---

Exercise 9.3   To consider your interactions with your partners

Take time to consider your interactions with your partners and answer the following questions:

1. What do I know about my partners' aspirations?

2. How do I as the junior partner fit into their plans?

3. Am I fulfilling the role that they expect of me?

4. Do I regard myself as equal to them in the partnership?

5. Do they regard me as equal to them in the partnership?

6. Am I fully involved in partnership decisions? If not, why not?

---

energy, changing too much too quickly saps our energy. When we are tired, we become irritable and make mistakes. Start with a well defined achievable project, in an area in which you are confident. A successful initial project will boost your confidence and raise the practice's opinion of your ability.

Set yourself a plan for the specific project:

1. Set a clear end point.

2. Identify a way of knowing when you have reached your goal.

3. Identify forces which will help you achieve your goal.

4. Identify forces which will work against you reaching your goal.

5. Define clear stages in reaching your goal, set a realistic time scale to each stage.

6. Review the project at a predetermined interval to check if successful.

Setting the pace of the change

It can be difficult, without building on experience, to judge how rapidly change can be introduced. If it is introduced too quickly there may be lack of understanding and resentment, if the introduction is too slow the practice team may become impatient. Probably the most important way of judging the speed at which the change can be introduced is to listen to the practice team. Listen to what they say and watch how they respond. It is helpful to have a trusted ally who will indicate if the pace is wrong:

Jane wanted to introduce a clinic for menopausal women. She sought the support of her female partner whom she knew would be interested and discussed her proposals with her. The two of them discussed their ideas at a practice meeting. The partnership was supportive. The two doctors undertook an audit of the care of women aged 45 to 60. With the practice manager, they identified a receptionist and practice nurse who would be responsible for assisting with the clinic and involved them in structuring the protocol. The four people set a date by which they hoped to be up and running. The receptionist and Jane talked over their ideas with the administrative staff. When they were ready, they presented their final plans to the whole practice. There were a few minor suggestions before advertising to the patients and implementation in three months. After six months Jane sought patients' and practice staff's views on the clinic.

Discussion: Jane set herself clear objectives, she discussed her plans with those concerned, involving all members of the practice. She audited the project to check that the results of her change were benefitting the practice.

Dealing with resistance to change

Not all of us will have such a successful project as Jane. Any project involving change may meet with a variety of resistors. Typical forms of human resistance are:

- parochial self interest
- misunderstanding and lack of trust
- different assessments of the situation and the proposed solution
- low tolerance of change.

It is important to identify the type of resistance which is likely to be met and select a strategy to deal with it. Table 9.1 identifies methods for dealing with resistance to change. The strategies that are identified are:

- education and communication
- participation and involvement
- facilitation and support
- negotiation and agreement
- manipulation and cooption
- implicit and explicit coercion.

Each situation will need a different solution depending on the nature of resistance and the timescale for implementation of the project. It is important to identify the nature of the resistance as early as possible and plan for it.

Rodgers[4] has described the diffusion of innovation. He suggests that those people who are most likely to be receptive to change are those who have been innovators in the past. Attempts to introduce change to other groups will take longer. Using this concept you may find that there is another member of the practice, not necessarily a partner, who is willing to accept your ideas for innovation and work with them. Once this has happened, other members of the practice are likely to take them up:

The Happy Valley Practice wanted to become a training practice. Dr Smart went on the local trainers' course and came back filled with enthusiasm. However, before he could be considered as a trainer the practice needed to summarize all its medical records. Dr Smart set out a timetable for the four partners to work with the administrative staff. He planned to have all the records summarized and on the computer within twelve months. After six months he reviewed their progress. The three younger partners were dismayed to find that Dr Large, the senior partner, had made very little progress. When asked why he pointed out that as he had been in the practice for thirty years he knew all the patients and their past histories and as he was retiring he could see no benefit in using his leisure time summarizing records. The younger partners understood his feelings and agreed that they should take on his records.

Discussion: There was no benefit in the change for Dr Large. Unfortunately, the other partners failed to recognize it in their eagerness.

Looking after the staff

At times we get swept along with our excitement for progress. Flushed with success, we look around for new areas to tackle. When a project has been completed take time to enjoy it and, in particular, take time to praise your staff

Table 9.1 Methods for dealing with resistance to change

Approach	Commonly used in situations	Advantages	Drawbacks
Education and communication	Where there is lack of information or inaccurate information and analysis.	Once persuaded, people will often help with the implementation of the change.	Can be very time consuming if lots of people are involved.
Participation and involvement	Where the initiators do not have all the information they need to design the change, and where others have considerable power to resist.	People who participate will be committed to implementing change and any relevant information they have will be integrated into the change plan.	Can be very time consuming if participants design an inappropriate change.
Facilitation and support	Where people are resisting because of adjustment problems.	No other approach works as well with adjustment problems.	Can be time consuming and expensive and still fail.
Negotiation and agreement	Where someone or some group will clearly lose out in a change, and where that person or group has considerable power.	Sometimes it is a relatively easy way to avoid major resistance.	Can be too expensive in many cases if it alerts others to negotiate for compliance.
Manipulation and cooption	Where other tactics will not work or are too expensive.	It can be a relatively quick and inexpensive solution to resistance problems.	Can lead to future problems if people feel manipulated.

From Kotter, J. P. and Schlesinger, L. A. Choosing strategies for change. In (Mayon White, B., ed.) *Planning and managing change*. London: Harper and Row, 1979.

for their contribution. If you have not been the prime mover in the change management but have been a supporter of the project, take time to record your and the practice's thanks to those concerned.

LEADERSHIP

In the first section of this book, we reflected on the history of general practice. Certain individuals within our profession set a clear vision for the future and forged ahead, sometimes at personal cost, to achieve their goal. Leadership is a topic that causes embarrassment among general practitioners, perhaps because we do not come from a hierarchial structure. We are reticent to put ourselves forward into leadership positions. Yet when we consider some of the practices around us that are struggling, it is often due to lack of leadership. A leader does not need to be an authoritarian figure. Effective leaders will have the skills to motivate the people that they work with, they possess the ability to scan the horizon for future developments and are preparing their practice for change before it arrives.

Leadership in general practice may depend on several factors; many of us still assume that the senior partner should take the lead role. In other partnerships a charismatic figure may take over; in others there may be a democratic election. Preferably, leadership will be sapiential, earned through respect of knowledge and ability. If the leadership of a practice is insecurely based, there is likely to be unhappiness and resentment. Good leadership depends not only on the individual but also on the other members of the group. It is likely that a practice will have different leaders for different tasks, individuals assuming responsibility for defined areas of the practice. Difficulties may arise when two or more individuals are vying for the lead role for a single task. Effective communication is essential when managing change in a partnership. Meetings with clear minutes that have been agreed by all concerned should help to avoid conflict.

SUMMARY

Managing change in practice can be great fun when it works well. It is important to have a clear plan of the proposed change, with a well-defined end point. Effective communication is essential, with all those concerned with the change being consulted. There is always likely to be resistance to change; if this can be identified early and handled in an appropriate way the project is more likely to be successful. Coping with change can be exhausting, when the project is finished there needs to be praise for all those concerned. Finally, we are not always successful, but we can always learn. When we are not successful in implementing change we need to take time to consider what we should do differently next time.

REFERENCES

1. Collings, S. General practice in England today. *Lancet*, 1950, **1**: 555–85.
2. What Sort of Doctor Working Party. *What sort of Doctor?* Report from general practice 23. London: Royal College of General Practitioners, 1985.
3. RCGP. *Fellowship by assessment.* Occasional paper 50. Royal College of General Practitioners, 1990.
4. Rodgers, E. M. *The diffusion of innovations* (3rd ed.). The Free Press, 1983.
5. Kotter, J. P. and Schlesinger, L. A. Choosing strategies for change. In (Mayon White, B., ed.) *Planning and managing change.* London: Harper and Row, 1979.

10 Education

It can be difficult for a new principal to find their way around the maze of postgraduate medical education. It seems as though there is a wealth of opportunities for learning of varying quality and relevance; fitting it into the average general practitioner's day can seem impossible. Each of us has to identify a way of keeping up to date with clinical knowledge while refining our skills, both clinical and managerial, and learning new skills. This, on top of a busy clinical day, may lead to encroachment on our personal lives.

PREPARING FOR POSTGRADUATE EDUCATION

The transition from registrar to young principal

During the training year there is likely to have been considerable emphasis on the transition from hospital doctor to general practitioner; the skills needed for working in an environment where the task was to minimize uncertainty are very different from those where we have to learn to live with uncertainty and minimize risk. Perhaps one of the biggest transitions that we have to make is that from registrar to principal in general practice. We have to learn to adapt from an environment which is equipped with tools and people to assist learning to one where we need to establish our own mechanisms to identify what we need to learn and then find a suitable way of learning it.

It may help to reflect on the task that your trainer undertook when he or she was helping you. Each trainer works with a blueprint of the knowledge, skills, and values that a registrar needs on completion of training. If a registrar is not matching up to that blueprint the trainer has difficulty signing the statement of satisfactory completion. The trainer takes the registrar through a series of situations early in the year to establish their current knowledge, skills and values; he then sets out with them a programme of learning to take the registrar from the current state to the blueprint. Most registrars will be aware that the trainer checks their progress through that programme as the year passes. Sometimes the progression is smooth, at other times there needs to be slight adjustments made to the programme as assessments identify deficiencies. At the same time the trainer will be aware of the areas that the registrar wants to cover, their preferred style of learning, and the things that motivate them. Principals in general practice need to develop the skills to identify their own 'blueprint' and then design a programme of learning to achieve it. They also need to develop mechanisms to check if they are moving towards their planned objective, to identify the things that motivate them, and to recognize their preferred ways of learning.

Exercise 10.1   To identify a learning plan

1. Write down five qualities you think would be the hallmark of an excellent general practitioner.

2. Write down how you think you match up to those qualities.

3. Write down how you decided how good you were.

    e.g. Feedback from partners, staff, or patients

        Feedback from colleagues, e.g. other young principals

        Self assessment through video, computer assessment, audit, etc.

        Previous feedback, e.g. from Trainer or Course Organizer

---

Aiming for excellence

In Chapter 12 we cover how to set a strategic plan for a practice and how individuals can work within that framework to set and monitor their own standards of care. Exercise 10.1 demonstrates one way of setting out a learning plan; it may seem tedious to commit it to paper but it is a very good discipline as it means that you have a written record which you can use for reference.

The principles of adult learning

Before you identify your own curriculum for the early years in your practice it might help to understand a little about adult learning. Adult learners are in a continuing process of growth and development, and they will want to build on previous experience. If the provider of education is unclear where the learner is on the developmental curve the education may be aimed at the wrong level. All adult learners bring with them previous experience and values, they are usually clear what they want to learn and how they will learn it. Adults have competing interests for their time—they may only be able to devote a relatively short period of time to learning and they will become irritated if learning is not effective. Most adults have developed a preferred learning style, which they will find difficult to change.

Adults learn about the world and about themselves through reflection on past action. They construct future action from reflections on their learning. Kolb described this as a cycle of experiential learning (Fig. 10.1). The learning process has been expanded by Pedlar *et al.* (Fig. 10.2): observation and reflection on experience leads to increased understanding; understanding in turn leads to insights, which allow development of new plans and new ways of behaving; the plans lead to action which stimulates the cycle.

Each of us has a preferred learning style. Honey and Mumford[1] described four learning styles, relating to each stage of Kolb's learning cycle. *Activists* like

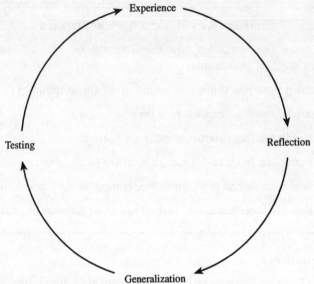

Fig. 10.1. The Kolb learning cycle. (From McGill, I. and Beaty, L. Action learning—a practitioner's guide. Kogan Page, 1992.)

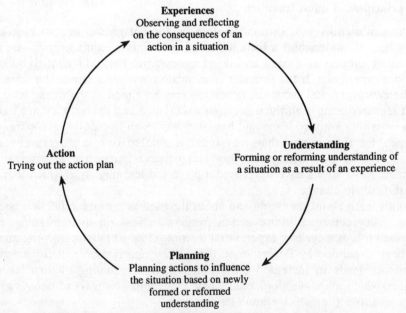

Fig. 10.2. The learning process. (From Pedlar *et al*. In: Action learning—a practitioner's guide. Ed. McGill, I. and Beaty, L. Kogan Page, 1992.)

to be exposed to new ideas and experiences. *Reflectors* prefer to reflect on the implication of the information presented. *Theorists* like to assimilate the new material and incorporate it with previous experiences. *Pragmatists* like to try out new knowledge. If pragmatists are placed in a lecture they are likely to become bored, wanting to try out the new information, similarly theorists feel uncomfortable working with a new idea before they have had time to assimilate it.

Tools to identify gaps in knowledge and skills

It can be difficult to identify what you don't know that you don't know, and it is perhaps one of the most challenging aspects of general practice. In hospital medicine there is a culture of identifying areas where there is lack of knowledge. In the training year continuous assessment usually identifies areas of weakness but many practices have yet to adopt a culture of constructive criticism. As a partner in a practice there may be instances where you suspect that another member of the team has a knowledge gap or is not confident in performing certain tasks; certainly recent media coverage of general practitioners' inability to take cervical smears causes concern about our ability to criticise our peers.

In practices where there is a culture of case discussion and observation of each others' work there may be no difficulty for a new principal. If the discussion is helpful rather than judgemental a new person should soon adapt, bringing to the discussion their own experiences. If a practice has yet to develop a culture of peer review the new partner has the choice of introducing it or seeking a similar process outside the practice. Going outside the practice may have benefits. It may be difficult for a younger doctor to openly comment adversely on a senior colleague's performance but it will have negative aspects too. It may be possible to bring to an outside group only those aspects of our work in which we feel confident, thereby failing to recognize our weaknesses:

Jane joined the Market Street Practice soon after completing her training. Before her interview she had been invited to meet the partners in their weekly lunch-time meeting. After she joined the practice she realized the importance of these meetings where the partners discussed a variety of clinical issues, often relating to difficult patients or recent journal articles. Jane enjoyed the feedback and soon realized that it was easy for her to make suggestions and constructive criticisms about patient care. Peter, a trainee from her group, had joined a neighbouring practice. Although the partners met weekly to discuss management issues there was little opportunity in the week to discuss clinical care. Peter missed the stimulation from the trainee group, so when he next met Jane he suggested that they should form a young principals' discussion group.

Discussion: Both doctors recognized that they needed a forum for discussing clinical issues. Jane was able to secure it through the practice, where constructive feedback was part of the culture. Peter sought it outside the practice. Both are equally useful although Jane had a forum where she was also able to comment on her partners' care.

Audit is perhaps the most important tool for identifying gaps in knowledge and skills. Table 10.1 sets out some areas where audit will identify areas of need. Some practices are moving into regular appraisal for all members of the

Table 10.1   Areas where audit might identify gaps in knowledge or skills

Audit	Areas identified
Review of referral letters	To assess the correlation between the referral diagnosis and the consultant opinion may reveal gaps in knowledge
Systematic review of the management of chronic diseases	To identify variations between partners in managing patients with chronic disease
Setting protocols for the management of chronic diseases	To identify new ideas on current practice and agree on a practice standard
Significant event analysis	To allow the whole practice to reflect in depth on individual patient care
Review of consultations recorded on video-tape	Allows the partners to observe and discuss consultation styles as well as giving observation of patient management

practice, including the partners. This should be a time where the partners can discuss openly areas where improvements need to be made. Each of us will have our own agenda for learning, but if a practice is going to develop and if we are to be part of that development, our individual learning needs will need to relate to the general direction of the practice.

THE POSTGRADUATE MEDICAL EDUCATION STRUCTURE

The postgraduate centre

The postgraduate centre used to be the focus of medical education, and in many areas it continues to fulfill that function. In most regions, the General Practice Tutor is based in the postgraduate centre. All postgraduate centres will have a selection of books and journals—if your centre does not stock an important journal, the GP Tutor may be able to advise the postgraduate committee to purchase it. Most postgraduate centres have sophisticated search facilities for identifying references; many also have a store of video-tapes and learning material which might be used for practice based learning. Probably the most important function of the centre remains that of a meeting place for general practitioners and hospital consultants. In the centre they are able to discuss patients informally.

The GP Tutor

General Practice Tutors are responsible for continuing medical education for general practitioners in the district; they work closely with the Postgraduate

Tutor and the Medical Audit Advisory Group. They are responsible for seeking the views of local practitioners regarding continuing medical education and ensuring that suitable events are held in the district. Many GP Tutors have a younger doctor working alongside them who takes responsibility for co-ordinating education for young principals. The GP Tutors are part of the postgraduate network. The name of your local tutor can be found through the postgraduate centre or through the Regional Adviser in General Practice's office.

The Regional Adviser in General Practice

Regional Advisers in General Practice are general practitioners who have a part time or full time appointment with the university to supervise postgraduate education for general practitioners. They work with a team of Associate Regional Advisers, Course Organizers and GP Tutors. Most young principals will have been in contact with a Regional Adviser in order to secure a Joint Committee Certificate. The Regional Adviser is responsible for recognizing educational activity for the postgraduate education allowance, which is usually administered through the GP Tutor network. Most Regional Advisers are concerned that the educational needs of young principals are not being met and many are actively seeking to redress the problem.

Prolonged study leave

The prolonged study leave is part of the Statement of Fees and Allowances. It is intended to give general practitioners an opportunity to work outside their practice, developing their skills. It is now available for full time or part time study. Prolonged study leave may be granted for personal study but the area chosen should be of benefit to general practice as a whole. One area for which it may be used in the early years in practice is to study for a higher degree such an an MSc. Applications are made to the Postgraduate Dean who will usually discuss them with the Regional Adviser in General Practice. All applications are then sent to the Department of Health, and those which receive the support of the Postgraduate Dean may be viewed more favourably. Applications should follow a logical format, similar to any application for funding. The application should identify not only how the proposed study will benefit the individual doctor but also how it will help the whole of the profession. A successful applicant should expect to submit a report at the end of the study period.

OPPORTUNITIES FOR LEARNING

The practice as a learning centre

Throughout this section there has been reference to the importance of a practice culture of learning and development. A practice which has an atmosphere of constructive criticism, where all members of the practice team are willing to point out areas for improvement, is likely to be one which will go forward. Such a practice will encourage time out from clinical responsibilities to refine and develop skills, particularly those which will bring areas of growth to the practice. The practice team may identify areas where all members of the team need to learn or be updated, such as cardio-pulmonary resuscitation or there may be specific areas for individuals:

The town centre practice undertook an audit of referral of patients to the skin outpatients. They were surprised to find how many patients they were referring with simple hand warts or verrucae. Philip, the newest recruit to the partnership, was particularly interested in dermatology. He suggested that he attend the dermatology clinic for a few weeks to brush up his skills and then introduce a 'wart clinic' in the practice.

   Discussion: The whole practice recognized the problem of high referrals in one area. One partner decided to update his skills to meet the need within the practice.

Working with a mentor

One of the transitions that a young principal may need to make when moving from being a registrar to becoming a principal in general practice is working without the trainer as a mentor. Those registrars who have worked with a trainer who was able to provide support without over-directing, to give feedback without being judgemental, and to encourage them to work to the limits of their capabilities, will probably be missing the trainer more than most. Many may be continuing the relationship.

   A good trainer becomes a mentor to the registrar, he will encourage the registrar to develop and to find out gaps in knowledge and skills, he will be around to discuss difficult ethical issues, and he will share the progress which is being made. Many trainers continue as a mentor beyond the training year, but many young principals may want to cultivate a new relationship. Although it is perfectly possible to work without a mentor, many of us find it helpful to relate to an individual and consult with them. As we progress through our professional lives we may find that we relate to more than one person, or we may change mentors as our needs alter.

Portfolio learning

Medicine has taken from the arts the concept of a portfolio of activity to demonstrate educational development. This concept fits particularly well for general practice, where there is a need for broad based activity, and a tendency to concentrate on the familiar. The learner identifies areas where there are knowledge or skill deficits and then identifies a series of activities to meet the perceived need. These might include attending courses, reading, using distance learning material, or membership of action learning groups. It is important to be specific about the aims of each activity. This will mean defining in detail the knowledge and skills which need to be learned. If this process is insufficiently detailed, it may be difficult to establish whether the objectives have been achieved. An important component of portfolio learning is the presence of a mentor, who will reflect with the learner on what has been achieved and what remains to be learned.[2] The mentor may be another general practitioner, or a member of the practice team:

Philip was interested in a discussion at the postgraduate centre on portfolio learning. After the meeting he asked the GP Tutor if he could try it out. The GP Tutor identified a local GP who was interested in medical education who was willing to act as Philip's mentor. Together, Philip and his mentor identified the main areas to be covered in the next twelve months and agreed a timetable. Philip's mentor offered to lend Philip some books on practice management to help. They agreed to meet again in eight weeks to assess progress.

Learning sets

A learning set is a term adopted from adult education. It consists essentially of a group of people who are all engaged in similar activities. The group meets regularly to discuss their progress. Through discussion, sharing of views, and reflection on how each member of the group has handled the task, the group learns how to undertake the task more effectively. A learning set usually has a group leader who understands the nature of the task, and who will help the group to maintain direction:

Five practices in the county were preparing for fundholding. The five lead partners and the five practice managers agreed that they would meet fortnightly to discuss the introduction of fundholding. The FHSA helped them identify a suitable group leader to work with them. Each member of the group agreed to share ideas and progress with the whole group.

Young practitioner groups

Balint, perhaps, described the first learning set of general practitioners.[3] The early groups explored the doctors' feelings about their patients, and reflected on the effect on the patients' management. In the early 1980s, general practitioners emerging from vocational training missed the support of their trainee group, many continued to meet to discuss areas of concern; sometimes the discussions related to clinical care, sometimes to management or personality issues. Most areas have a group of young doctors who meet regularly, usually about once a month. The name of the convener of a local group can usually be obtained from the postgraduate centre or GP Tutor.

Skills training

Most young principals have had experience of training in consultation skills. Although this might be an area where they have reasonable confidence, the consultation is the cornerstone of general practice and no matter how good we believe that we are there is always something more to be learned.

Practice management is often an area which receives less rigorous attention during training. There are important areas of knowledge which may need to be plugged but probably more important are those skills which relate to the management of people, especially negotiating skills, assertiveness skills, appraisal skills, interviewing, and selection skills. There has been extensive coverage of these areas for fundholding practices but, unfortunately, often the new partner is not able to benefit. The Women's Unit, a unit within the Department of Health with responsibility for developing management skills in women in the health service, has been especially keen to promote training in these areas:

Susan was finding working in a practice as a part-time partner difficult. She felt that she was not fully involved in practice decisions although she regularly attended all the meetings. The final straw came when she heard that the registrar was to have her room and that she should use whichever room was spare. She spoke to the local GP Tutor who suggested that she might benefit from assertiveness training. He identified a local course for her. Susan was surprised at the effect of the course which gave her confidence to put her point across to the partners.

Updating courses

There is a plethora of activities to update clinical knowledge, varying from a week on the Nile to the weekly postgraduate lecture. Many of these events also cover updates on knowledge of practice management, including financial and tax information.

Distance learning

Since the introduction of the Postgraduate Education Allowance there has been an expansion in the number of distance learning packages. Some require very little activity and are not likely to result in dramatic changes in practice, others, however, are extremely well written, are often associated with 'summer schools' and may result in a certificate. Some of the distance learning packages are very suitable to be used as in-house training material for the practice. A full list of distance learning packages approved for the Postgraduate Education Allowance is available from the GP Tutor:

Mark had a young family, his wife worked and they found it difficult if either of them had to spend the night away from home. Mark wanted to develop his management skills. After discussion with the GP Tutor he identified a suitable distance learning course which he could do in the evenings while the children were young.

Reading

Some doctors find reading an important method of keeping up to date, others find it less effective. It can be difficult to decide what to read when so much comes through the door. As well as the refereed journals and the free medical press, there is information from the Department of Health and the FHSA. It is important for all of us to be aware of progress and to organize reading in a way that minimizes the risk of overlooking major medical breakthroughs. Each of us needs to organize our reading; trying to scan major journals such as the British Medical Journal and the Journal of the Royal College of General Practitioners whilst updating ourselves with review articles in Update or the Practitioner. The free medical press can be useful for keeping abreast of political events, but they cannot substitute for the academic literature.

There is now a wealth of books relating to general practice. Most trainees will have become familiar with many of the classic texts during their training year. There are many books relating to management and adult education that are relevant for much of our work. It may be useful to reflect on how you use books and the place of the practice library. We are familiar with using a book to look up a clinical condition, often we might refer to two or more texts to seek alternative views. Many management and general practice texts can be used in the same way:

Roger was thinking about introducing staff appraisal. He had been on a workshop and felt confident that he had the ability. His practice manager was keen but was not confident, she preferred to let Roger take the lead. Roger asked to borrow some of her management books and together they prepared a proforma for conducting the appraisal interview and another for giving feedback.

Practices vary in the books that they hold. Some have a few books in each surgery, others have an extensive catalogued library, including videotapes. Exercise 10.2 offers one way of reflecting on your practice library.

Higher degrees

There has been a proliferation of higher degrees relating to general practice, ranging from the diploma in dermatology to an MBA. Most of the courses preparing for the higher degree are structured and very well organized. Each will offer a range of skills which can be learned. Some can be taken through distance learning.

Many universities are now offering taught MSc courses in general practice. These courses are designed to give a broad research approach to general

---

Exercise 10.2   To identify the content of a practice library

1. What books does your practice have?

2. How are they used?

3. What books and journals would it be useful to have in the practice?

practice, many are multidisciplinary. The content varies with the university. The courses may be full time or part time. Current training for general practice does not equip the doctors with research skills, unlike most other specialities, so these courses which are designed to enhance research skills are highly valued. Although all general practitioners need to understand research methodology and be able to evaluate a paper not all will want to spend time actively engaged in research (as opposed to audit). Many general practitioners have now completed an MSc course and have found it extremely useful:

Mary had been a partner in her practice for five years. She thought that she would like to become a Course Organiser but before she did she wanted to be clear that she understood research methodology. She went to the Regional Adviser in General Practice who suggested that she consider an MSc course. Mary wrote for prospectuses and decided that it would be best for the practice if she opted for a part time course. She sought further advice in relation to prolonged study leave and with support from the Regional Adviser she wrote an application which was successfully funded.

Higher professional training

Many regions are now providing structured education for young principals. The training varies with each region, some consist of residential modules with group activity between modules, others are based on a regular weekly half day. The course content should reflect the concerns of the participants, often there will be considerable focus on relationships and communication:

Tariq wanted to be a trainer. He knew that the practice would have to adjust some of the ways in which it worked but he was not confident that he had the knowledge and skills to lead the changes. He discussed his difficulties with the local Course Organiser who suggested that he apply for a place on the regional higher professional training programme.

The role of the FHSA in education

Many FHSAs are actively involved in educating general practitioners, particularly those who are fundholding. They may provide management training for general practitioners and their staff. The FHSA has a staff training budget which could be useful if a practice is undertaking high level in-house training.

SUMMARY

Education in general practice often does not follow a logical path from identifying practice direction to practice aims and training needs. It is important that valuable time spent on education takes the practice and the individual forward in the intended direction. It is important that each member of the team identifies major areas where they want to update their skills. Young principals often have difficulty with the personnel management skills, which could be met through a variety of local activities.

REFERENCES

1. Honey, P. and Mumford, A. *The manual of learning styles*. London: Peter Honey, 1984.
2. RCGP: Royal College of General Practitioners, 1993. *Portfolio-based learning in general practice*. Occasional paper 63.
3. Balint, H. *The doctor, his patient and the illness*. London: Pitman Medical, 1964.

11 Stress and the health of doctors

A lifetime in general practice can be a daunting prospect. Coping with patients and their families, living in the community, managing a practice can all take their toll if young practitioners do not set up and maintain systems to protect their own health. General practitioners, like other health professionals, often give little regard to their own health. However, like all other members of society, we too are susceptible to illness and need to ensure that we place ourselves in a position to receive appropriate medical care. As this book is written primarily for young general practitioners, and as this group seem to suffer stress related illnesses more than other illnesses, this chapter focuses mainly on the causes of stress and how they might be relieved.

As a doctor joins a new partnership there is often nothing further from their mind than their own health. When it comes to choosing a general practitioner for themselves and their families it is easy to select one of their own partners. This may work well initially, life is busy enough without having to find time to keep an appointment with a local practitioner for renewal of a repeat prescription, or for treatment of minor illness in the family, but it can be very difficult to advise a partner about their own health.

General practitioners are particularly susceptible to depression and abuse of drugs, including alcohol. The incidence of suicide in doctors is 3.5 times higher than in the general population. The reasons for this are not clear, but it is easy to speculate about the effect of the job and the access to information about suicide.

When a general practitioner does become ill it can be very difficult to respond normally to the illness. There is a tendency for self-referral to a specialist, often informally without reference to a general practitioner. This may not cause too many problems when the illness is physical but, as we are all aware, many patients present with physical symptoms when the cause of the illness is stress or unhappiness. If depression and stress related illnesses are not recognized by a young doctor it may be detrimental to him, his family, and his patients. Much of the rest of this chapter focuses on the cause of stress and ways of coping, but perhaps the most important message is to register yourself and your family with a local general practitioner, outside the partnership, and consult that doctor as you would want to be consulted.

FACTORS THAT CREATE STRESS

Each of us will respond differently to various situations. Some of us will find new and uncertain circumstances exciting and stimulating, others will find them difficult to handle. Life might be very dull without some challenging aspects to it but with too many we become anxious and distressed. The early years in general practice are likely to be packed with new situations; as well as settling into a practice the young principal is likely to have many significant life events. A house move, marriage, pregnancy, and young children all add their burden and compound an already stressful situation.

Young principals find providing out of hours care, particularly through the night, difficult to cope with; they also find that they lack the skills to manage and respond to change. Both these situations are most significant. Traditionally, the new partner has been expected to contribute to out of hours care, while those nearer retirement may be relieved of the burden. Some practices still follow lifelong patterns of the junior partner covering Friday night, prolonging the ordeal of the weekend cover. Many practices look to the new partner to bring them up to date. Some are asking a partner straight from training to take a lead role in fundholding. Others may expect a new partner to take a major role in audit or health promotion. At the interview these ideas may seem exciting and indeed, with the appropriate level of support and cooperation from others in the practice, the tasks may be stimulating and challenging. If, between the interview and starting in the practice there have been other life events, and if the partnership does not give the expected support, these activities may prove too much.

STRESS AND THE CONSULTATION

Many general practitioners find consultations stressful. Young practitioners are concerned in particular about their level of clinical knowledge and skills. This seems to be particularly important when caring for friends or colleagues. General practice can be very lonely, particularly when there is no practice ethos of discussing clinical problems. When the patient with the difficult problem is also a friend or colleague, confidentiality may preclude discussion with other people such as fellow young principals or spouse.

The heartsink patient has been described recently. Our training has often created in us an expectation that patients get better and most of our training takes place in the hospital where we have the opportunity to discharge patients who do not have physical disease. The year in the training practice shields us from many of the chronically sick patients.[1] The new principal in general practice will often encounter 'heartsink patients' for the first time; if there are no opportunities to discuss these patients, either within the partnership or in a discussion group, anxiety begins to develop, and fear that perhaps serious illness is being missed.

Howie and others have found other stress provoking situations in the working day. Probably the most significant of these was the stress created in some doctors when they were expected to consult more rapidly than the rate at which they felt comfortable.[2] All too frequently we hear training practices talk about preparing the trainee for the 'real world' which they believe hinges on the five minute consultation, yet in reality most of us feel very uncomfortable working at this speed for prolonged periods. None of us likes to run late in our surgeries, and we become more anxious if we are behind schedule and have other external pressures such as a partner waiting to use the room or a meeting to get to.

General practitioners seem more stressed since the introduction of the 1990 contract. We have certainly been asked to increase our activity and take on new responsibilities; and there is more administrative work. Some practices coped better with the imposed changes than others. The ability to cope with the changes seemed to be related to the level of organization, with better organized practices, in particular training practices, faring better. Finally, just as an unhappy marriage is stressful so too is an unhappy partnership. Where there is rivalry and resentment between partners conflict arises, often focusing on inequalities in workload and profit share.

RECOGNITION OF STRESS

A certain element of anxiety can be helpful. If we are totally confident about our level of expertise in patient care we may lose the incentive to learn new skills and refresh our knowledge. Each day we are likely to encounter patients with new and puzzling symptoms. Many of us need this challenge to refer to our books and learn new facts and concepts. However, there comes a time when too many new situations become overwhelming with the resultant feeling of being unable to cope. Warning signs may include:

• irritability
• changes in sleeping, eating, and drinking patterns
• difficulty concentrating and taking decisions
• worrying or anger over trivial situations
• physical symptoms, with no organic basis, such as low back pain or headache.

Stressed doctors become carried along by too much to do, they leave no time for relaxation, and fall into an exhausted state.

WAYS OF COPING

Coping with stress falls into two broad strategies; there are general activities, many of which will be included in the advice that we give to patients, and there are specific problem solving activities.

General activities

It can be difficult as a new principal in general practice to cope with the demands of a new job, young family, and often a new environment and still leave time for leisure activities. Weekend sporting events may be disrupted by on call, evening activities may be difficult when there are late surgeries and on call. It is important to decide for yourself how best you relax, perhaps through music, physical activity, walking, gardening, going to the theatre or cinema, or spending time with friends and family. Regular aerobic, physical activity reduces anxiety by release of endorphins. As well as reducing stress, physical activity of this kind maintains a healthy cardiovascular system and helps to maintain body weight at a reasonable level. It is very easy to allow cigarette and alcohol consumption to increase when work is stressful. Alcohol, in particular, is frequently used by doctors, and rather than helping relieve stress it may contribute to it.

We are all familiar with patients who present in our surgeries with the effect of a surfeit of life events. By the very nature of being in the early years in partnership a young principal will have recently changed his or her job. With that job change there may have been financial expenditure associated with purchasing a building or equipment. The new partnership may also involve a move into the practice area. Many young doctors postpone marriage or starting a family until they are settled. Having found a partnership the new job may be followed shortly by a marriage or pregnancy. We have already identified two or more significant life events that will add to any stress of a new partnership.

Problem solving

Before identifying solutions for likely problems, it is beneficial to take time to identify the situations that are particularly stressful to you. Perhaps one of the most disturbing situations for all of us is the feeling of not being in control of our life. Many new principals in general practice feel that they do not have an equal voice in partnership decisions. Understandably, they find this difficult to handle, and they start to feel resentful. It can be difficult to join a partnership and influence it so that it moves towards your ideal practice, but the consequences of not doing so are serious.

You may find it helpful to consider the strategic planning exercise on p. 130. The exercise includes describing five aspects of your practice you would like to be cited for merit in a special reward. If you were able to work with your partners, you may now have a practice mission statement. The next stage of the exercise is to devise a plan that can be achieved over the next five years. Remember that you will not be able to achieve it all at once, pace yourself. There may be key points that are already clear to you, a practice manager or partner planning retirement, or a planned move in premises. Use these changes as opportunities. It is useful to prepare an individual plan, setting your own goals. Take time to do this now, following the same stages of:
1. set a vision
2. identify the current situation
3. identify the helping and hindering forces
4. write a plan
   (a) Be specific about each of your objectives.
   (b) Put a date by which each of your objectives can be achieved.
   (c) Be realistic; if you try to achieve too much too quickly you may become despondent.
   (d) Share your plan with someone whom you can trust to give you an honest opinion, a friend or spouse.

Exercise 11.1   To identify situations that make you feel stressed and those that make you feel satisfied

1. Over the next full week try to be more aware of your own feelings, in particular when you feel anxious and when you feel well or elated.

2. Keep a diary, write down the factors that led to your feelings. Try to be as explicit as possible.

3. Continue to record in your diary at home. At the end of the week take time to look through your diary.

4. Discuss your conclusions with someone who knows you well, perhaps your spouse or a close friend. Have they noticed you becoming tense in similar situations to the ones you describe?

5. Spend time thinking about the factors that make you feel good. Are any of them at work, if so, look for common patterns?

6. Place each of your factors that make you anxious into two groups, those that you can influence and those that seem beyond your control.

Your strategic plan is something that you should refer to regularly. Being in control and planning for change helps reduce stress. At this point it may be useful to refer back to your list of factors which you found stressful. How many of them will be reduced or removed if you can achieve your action plan? There remain several situations that seem to make young principals anxious, taking the fun out of general practice.

OUT-OF-HOURS WORK

It seems likely that out of hours responsibility will remain part of general practice in the foreseeable future. Most of us have been frightened visiting at night; emphasis has been placed on women general practitioners, but there are risks for both sexes. Night work also makes us tired and, when the visits are requested without regard for the welfare of the doctor concerned, we become resentful. Out-of-hours work is certainly a topic frequently discussed by most general practitioners. It may be an important topic to raise at your next practice meeting. Do the other partners feel the same way as you? Would a practice mobile telephone help, without creating major expenditure? Should the practice be thinking about patient education regarding the use of the doctor at night? Would a later evening surgery reduce the early evening calls? Would using a deputizing service relieve some of the pressure, particularly for the middle of the night calls? Is there opportunity to join a local co-operative?

Exercise 11.2 To enhance the enjoyable aspects of your day

1. Turn to your list of situations that made your feel content or pleased (exercise 11.1).

2. Are you able to create additional similar situations in your week?

3. Were there tasks on your list which you enjoyed but which other partners seemed to find irksome? Could you offer to trade some of the tasks that you find difficult for this group?

4. Could you adapt your use of time to allow opportunity for more leisure activities that you enjoy?

CLINICAL CONFIDENCE

All of us like to feel that we are providing optimum care. Sometimes our standards may be compromised through lack of time, and sometimes through lack of ability. When this happens, we feel uncomfortable. This can be particularly difficult for a new entrant to general practice, training for our speciality is the shortest of all medical specialities, yet we are expected to have the broadest range of knowledge and skills.

General practice is also one of the few specialities that lack organized higher professional training, so most of us are continuing to learn in the post. There are people around to help. Most districts have an active young principals group. These groups address a wide range of issues, many focus on managing change. However, if other members of the group are also concerned about clinical skills there may be an opportunity to spend time with a consultant or senior registrar thinking through and discussing clinical situations. It may be possible to learn new skills such as joint injection, or improve old ones such as consultation skills.

COPING WITH A COMPLAINT

There has been considerable media coverage on our current complaints system. Having a complaint made against you is still seen as a sign of failure, even before the complaint is heard. Most complaints still relate to a breakdown in communication between patient and doctor. Trying to avoid a complaint may lead to defensive medicine, which usually results in poor patient care. Some cultures positively welcome complaints, feeling that it helps them to modify their practices to suit their customer. It is unlikely that British general practice will go to these lengths but the introduction of an informal complaints procedure, involving the practice manager, may give patients a forum for expressing dissatisfaction without the negative effect of involving the FHSA:

Mr Brown rang for a late visit for his three years old daughter. Susan was the receptionist on duty that day. Immediately after she had taken the call, Dr Gruff rang her to say that he needed a cervical spatula urgently. Susan had to go to the treatment room for the spatula. When she returned to the desk she had forgotten the request for the visit. Dr Keen was on duty for the evening. Soon after he arrived home, Mr Brown rang to ask when he was coming to see his daughter. Dr Keen went straight round and saw the little girl. Mr Brown was understandably angry. Dr Keen reassured him that the matter would be taken up. The following morning Mr Brown asked the receptionist how to make a complaint. He was directed to the practice manager. The practice manager listened carefully to Mr Brown. She explained the practice procedure to identify what had happened and told him that she would contact him. The practice manager found out that Susan had been on duty the evening before. When she heard Susan's story, she was sympathetic but firm about the importance of recording visit requests. She made a note in Susan's file about the event. She brought the topic to the next practice meeting, where it was agreed that Dr Gruff should be more aware of the pressures on the receptionists and that there should be an identified member of staff who would be responsible for ensuring that the consulting rooms were fully stocked. The practice manager wrote to Mr Brown to explain the changes that had been made and invited him to discuss it further should he wish. Mr Brown was satisfied that the practice had addressed the problem.

Discussion: The practice had a procedure for handling complaints with which all the staff were familiar. The practice manager listened sympathetically to the complaint and then, without judgement, heard from the member of staff concerned. A record was made. Repeated errors by a member of staff may lead to disciplinary procedures. The whole practice team were able to discuss the problem. Relationships in the practice were sufficiently good that an austere doctor could be gently reprimanded, and changes made in the practice to reduce the risk of a receptionist leaving her desk.

Not all complaints are handled smoothly within the practice, some are taken to the FHSA or Health Board. Common reasons for complaints are:

- failure to visit
- failure to examine
- failure to diagnose
- failure to refer
- failure to treat

Patients and their relatives complain most frequently not because of doctor error but because the doctor did not do what was expected of them. Frightened or anxious patients find it difficult to give an accurate history, often creating an impatient doctor. If the doctor becomes aggressive or irascible it is soon transmitted to the patient and may result in a complaint. Perhaps we are at our most vulnerable when we visit at the end of evening surgery. Tired and hungry, we may be irritated by being asked to visit a patient who could easily have come to surgery. A simple solution may be that the practice should arrange for a hot drink and a biscuit for the duty doctor at the end of the day.

It is important to keep accurate records of patient contacts including telephone conversations. It may be up to thirteen weeks before the complaint is made. During this time our memories might fail us. If there is warning of a complaint do take time to write a detailed account of the event, and discuss the situation with your defence organization. Whatever happens, it is unacceptable to alter the patient records after the event:

Susan was the third doctor to see Mrs Young in a week. Mrs Young has been coughing for ten days, she had called out a partner the previous week and the duty doctor two nights before the consultation. Mrs Young appeared unwell, she was breathless and had a dry cough. Susan examined her carefully. She was surprised that the patient had no signs of pneumonia, despite the initial impression. Susan thought that it was likely that Mrs Young had mycoplasma pneumonia and started her on Erythromycin. Two days later, Susan received a letter from one of the local physicians.' He was a friend of the family and had been asked to see Mrs Young. When he had examined her he found a consolidated left lower lobe. He was arranging for her to have an X-ray and blood tests.

A week later a neighbouring GP rang because the Young family were asking to join his list. They were dissatisfied with the care that Susan had provided and they had told him they were going to complain because Susan had failed to make a correct diagnosis. Susan took photocopies of all the records before they were returned to the FHSA. Fortunately, the X-ray result came back to her showing patchy consolidation on the right and the blood tests confirmed mycoplasma infection. Susan rang her defence organization and talked the case through. It was only while she was discussing it that she realised that the X-ray had not supported the consultant's clinical findings and that she had acted correctly. Susan heard no more about a complaint.

Discussion: No matter how carefully we might feel that we treat patients there are always unexpected situations. Susan had kept accurate information on Mrs Young. She had prepared herself for a hearing should one arise. Neither the consultant nor the patient would appreciate the anguish that Susan went through during that time, which could have been avoided by the consultant observing ethical procedures.

STATUS IN THE PARTNERSHIP

British general practice is unusual in its system of instant partnerships. Although most practices have a probationary period, a young principal might expect to be a partner in a practice within six months, working to parity over two to three years. This usually gives the young doctor responsibility for a list of patients together with liability for the partnership. In return the junior partner might expect to be a full profit sharing partner within three years. However, this may be where equality ends. Although a full profit sharing partner should expect to have an equal say in partnership decisions the reality may be far from that situation. New principals feel that the practice is somehow beyond their control and they express a sense of helplessness about the direction of the partnership. This has been cited as a cause of dissatisfaction and stress by young principals. We hope that the chapter on managing change will help to identify some ways of altering the situation. Other solutions often rest in young principals' groups or additional managerial skills gained following the completion of vocational training.

COPING WITH PARTNERSHIP DISPUTES AND ILLNESS

Most partnerships have difficult patches; these can be extremely stressful. The most common areas for disagreement are profit shares and workload. The disagreement may rumble through the partnership, never really surfacing, or it may result in an open discussion. Where all partners work full time and take an equal profit share there may be little cause for concern. When one or more partners have outside commitments or work part time, conflict may arise. However, the solution may be simple:

Dr Busy liked to take her children to school. This made her twenty minutes late for the start of her morning surgery. The other partners drew her attention to the problem and together they agreed that she should start and finish her surgery twenty minutes later.

Or it may be extremely complex:

Dr Green had a heart attack two years before he was due to retire. He took three months sick leave from the practice and then returned full time. His two partners allowed him to ease back gently, continuing to take on his night work, and keeping his surgeries light. After six months there was no sign of Dr Green returning to normal nor recognizing that he should reduce his profit share. The crisis arose when holiday time came round, effectively leaving one partner, Dr Brown, covering the on call. After a week, Dr Brown's husband exploded, his wife was exhausted and there had been no recognition of her contribution by Dr Green. Dr Brown decided that when Dr Black returned from his holiday the partners would have to tackle the problem. She called a partnership meeting where Dr Black and Dr Brown set out the problem for Dr Green, who was extremely upset. He had hoped that after all his years in the practice that they would allow him to stay until retirement. The two younger doctors felt equally hurt. Together the three agreed some options for Dr Green to consider. Dr Green eventually opted, reluctantly, for early retirement.

Perhaps the hardest problem to deal with is a partner with psychiatric illness:

Dr Young had been in partnership with Dr Smith and Dr Bell for two years. Dr Smith worked part time. Dr Young had noticed that Dr Bell often went to the local pub on his way home, sometimes at lunch time too. At first, Dr Young was not aware that it was causing a problem, but soon he realized that Dr Bell often appeared aggressive in the afternoons. His worst suspicions were confirmed when Dr Bell was obviously drunk when he returned for the evening surgery. He managed to persuade Dr Bell to go home. He rang Dr Smith but received little support. Dr Young decided to confide in his ex-trainer, who listened carefully and suggested that Dr Young should first try to discuss the problem with Dr Bell. If that failed he might approach Mrs Bell or the Local Medical Committee (LMC).

After coffee the next day Dr Young asked to speak to Dr Bell in private. He referred to the evening surgery and asked if there was a problem. Dr Bell replied that it had been the landlord's birthday and that Dr Young should not get upset about one occasion. He apologized for the extra work it had put on Dr Young and offered to cover Dr Young's next Saturday surgery.

Two weeks later Mrs Bell came to the surgery looking for her husband. She saw Dr Young and asked if she might have a confidential word. She apologized for her husband's behaviour and then tearfully explained how concerned she was about the drinking. She asked Dr Young if he could persuade her husband to seek help. Dr Bell continued to refuse to acknowledge the problem drinking until he was stopped in his car and breathalysed.

Dr Young sought help from the Chairman of LMC. Together they made Dr Bell agree to see a psychiatrist and enter a treatment programme.

Discussion: It is extremely difficult to handle a partner's illness, particularly when it is psychiatric. One way of avoiding some of the difficulties is to insist that partners and their families are not registered with the practice. The LMC will usually help in partnership disputes or partnership illness.

MANAGING AND RESPONDING TO CHANGE

Perhaps the major expressed cause of dissatisfaction with general practice since the introduction of the NHS reforms has been the effect of imposed change. This seems to have had the same response on all general practitioners across the country. However, the consequence for young principals may have been more significant if they are expected to lead a practice in coping with the imposed changes, or if they have wanted to respond to the changes but find difficulty taking the practice with them.

REINFORCING THE POSITIVE ASPECTS OF GENERAL PRACTICE

This chapter has focused on the difficulties faced by young principals, which lead to feelings of an inability to cope. It may be helpful to reflect on the aspects of our lives which we find enjoyable and stimulating, it may be possible to increase these activities without creating additional workload. Audit is a tool that can be used to highlight where a practice is successful, either by monitoring one aspect of care, and possibly entering for doctor of the year award or by using significant event analysis to discuss successes as well as complaints.

WHERE TO GO FOR HELP

There may be times when all your strategies for maintaining your morale seem to fail, everything looks black. There are people around who will help. Most general practitioners have experienced the same feelings as you are enduring. One of the partners or a member of the staff, perhaps the practice manager, may lend a friendly ear and come up with some suggestions. Your spouse will know you well, and is likely to be prepared to listen. Try to locate a young principals' group soon after starting as a principal. Some trainees who have settled into local practices continue to meet. These groups provide a useful forum for discussing problems, perhaps those that cannot be aired in the partnership. Although you may not be a member or associate of the Royal College of General Practitioners, this group of doctors will also provide support. Our College is based on geographical faculties. Most faculties have a member of the faculty board who is responsible for the welfare of new principals. The Local Medical Committee has a responsibility for the welfare of practitioners in the area. The telephone number of the Secretary or Chairman can be obtained through the FHSA. There is a service which cares for sick doctors. The number can be obtained through your LMC or it is to be found in the advertisement section of the British Medical Journal. Most Trainers and Course Organizers are delighted to hear from past trainees. A telephone call or a visit may help to put your problem in perspective. Each district in the United Kingdom has a General Practice Tutor and Course Organiser (Associate Advisers in Scotland). This group of general practitioners is familiar with the problems encountered by new principals in general practice and will usually go out of their way to help. Their names can be obtained from the postgraduate centre or from the Regional Adviser in General Practice.

SUMMARY

Life in general practice can be stressful, each of us has a different tolerance of stressful situations. Partnerships which are working well reduce stress, there are many strategies which can be used to avoid partnership difficulties and stressful situations. Although our work is important, so is the doctor's health. Try to practise what you tell your patients about a healthy life-style. If things do go badly wrong there are many people about to help.

REFERENCES

1. Hasler, J. C. *Clinical experiences of trainees in general practice.* MD thesis. University of London, 1982.
2. Howie, J. G. R. Quality of caring—Landscapes and curtains. *Journal of the Royal College of General Practitioners*, 1987; **37**: 4–10.

12 Achieving quality in general practice

The 1990 contract raised awareness of audit in general practice. Medical Audit Advisory Groups (MAAGs) were set up and most practices set about the task of audit, some more enthusiastically than others. It was not until some years later that we reflected on what we were achieving. Although many practitioners were busy evaluating their care this was often isolated from the daily practice activity. The audits taking place were often not being used to take the practice forward.

Although there has been frequent reference to quality in primary care since the NHS reforms, we have few definitions of what is meant by quality. Quality is frequently associated with managerial concepts and when phrases such as *total quality management* and *continuous quality management* are used many practitioners are understandably irritated or bewildered. Quality control was a term introduced in America from Japan to ensure uniformity of factory production. The terminology has crept into management issues in British general practice and some practices are working towards BS5750, the British quality standard for industry. BS5750 is a concept devised for industry which measures consistency of quality but does not necessarily measure the performance of an organization against predetermined standards. General practice does not fit easily into the production model; although we might seek consistency in our management procedures we must work with individual patients and adapt our care to meet their needs and expectations. Much of the thinking about the consultation has been based on the premise that we will not achieve good care unless we recognize individual patient concerns and expectations.[1]

The threat of reaccreditation has focused our thoughts more acutely on what we understand by quality and how we might measure it. Some of the early work in defining good general practice was done through the Royal College of General Practitioners and published in *The report from general practice. What sort of doctor?*.[2] This document was designed to be used for assessment when visiting a practice. The purpose of the visit should be entirely educational with feedback to the practice on their strengths and weaknesses. The document sets out a series of statements under the broad headings of availability and accessibility, clinical competence, communication, and professional values. It outlines how the practice can be observed, team members interviewed, and conclusions drawn about care provided. The headings then form a basis of a report which is submitted to the practice.

Ten years on from *What sort of doctor?* there exist various models of assessing quality against a predefined standard. Perhaps the most common is the training practice visit. In some areas the MAAG has taken a lead and is encouraging practice appraisal. Nationally the gold standard is the Royal College of General Practitioners' Fellowship by Assessment.

WHAT IS GOOD QUALITY GENERAL PRACTICE?

We are often prevented from defining what we mean by good quality by the difficulty that we perceive in how others see us. How often have we heard members of our community comment 'He's a jolly doctor you know, sends you straight to hospital, no messing' and our managers say 'That's a good practice, low prescribing costs'. Rather than trying to define what we mean by good quality we are seduced into trying to conform to how we perceive others would want us to be. High quality health care is a difficult concept to manage, there are no easy measurements which can identify high quality easily. Prescribing is perhaps one area where high cost may be an indicator of high or low quality. When considering prescribing for respiratory disease, high cost prescribing may be an indicator of poor quality care but high cost prescribing in terms of inhaled steroids for treatment of asthma may indicate high quality care. What is important is that prescribing is appropriate, a concept which is difficult to measure.

There are, however, markers of a high quality practice and these often relate to organizational issues. A well organized practice has put itself in a position to deliver high quality clinical care, the same cannot be said for a poorly organized practice. There can be no practice or practitioner who would want to be thought of as providing sub-optimum care yet all of us are aware that we are not providing the best care for all of our patients all of the time. We may be limited by resources but more frequently we are hampered by our own processes.

In order for a practice to provide excellent care, the health care professionals should be achieving the expected professional standard supported by management systems to ensure that patients can gain access to the health care professional and that the information necessary to provide the clinical care is available. A practice which is providing good quality care could therefore be defined as one in which every member of the practice team is setting their own standards and monitoring their performance within an overall strategic framework to provide optimal patient care.

QUALITY IN CLINICAL CARE

General practice has been proud of the way in which the practice team can deliver care to the patients. There is considerable attention paid to team working skills in the training year, yet we rarely take time to reflect who is in the team and how they contribute to the care of patients:

The Town Centre Practice looked after more patients than usual with chronic mental conditions. All the staff felt uncomfortable because this group of patients seemed unable to use the practice properly and they seemed to receive less than adequate care. Dr Young decided to hold a practice meeting to discuss the problem. She invited all the practice administrative staff, the doctors, the practice nurse, the community psychiatric nurse, and the health visitor. After setting out the reason for the meeting the team discussed the level of care which they thought this group should receive. Dr Young then asked everyone to think about their individual role in achieving optimum care for the group.

The receptionists worked together. They agreed they should keep some appointments free each day to fit in patients with chronic mental illness; let the community psychiatric nurse know if one of this group failed to keep an appointment; achieve continuity of care by arranging appointments so that the patients were seen by only one or two doctors.

The practice nurse thought that she could offer to give routine Modecate injections once the patient was stabilized. This would free the community psychiatric nurse. She was also aware that this group did not attend health promotion clinics so she could take the opportunity to identify risk factors, in particular she might persuade some of the women to have a smear.

The community psychiatric nurse felt that he should be working more closely with the practice. He would arrange a time when he could discuss patients with the doctors each week.

The health visitor thought for a while. Although she cared for a few children whose parents had chronic mental illness, she had very little contact with most of the adults. She then realized that she could work with the carers, giving support and helping them to educate the patients in health issues.

The data clerk worked with the practice manager, together they considered ways of maintaining an accurate register of patients with chronic mental illness, including information about hospital follow-up and the date each patient was last seen by a doctor in the practice.

The doctors agreed that they should give continuity of care for patients with chronic mental illness. They agreed to work with the practice nurse to provide health promotion opportunistically. The doctors then agreed a range of first line medication and features which should prompt referral for the common major psychiatric conditions. Dr Brown had not had any formal training in psychiatry, he thought that an updating course would be useful to brush up his knowledge and skills.

Dr Young was delighted that each member of the practice team could make small adjustments to provide a better service for patients with chronic mental illness. She suggested that they should meet again in six months and that each member of the team should measure their current activity against the standard they had just set.

Discussion: The town centre practice spent an afternoon considering the care of their patients with chronic mental illness, they agreed a common goal and then set individual standards to reach the goal. They could use the same process to set standards for all the major chronic diseases, perhaps most importantly each member of the practice team was able to take pride in doing a job well, raising morale in the practice.

QUALITY IN PRACTICE MANAGEMENT

Although most general practitioners would agree that their prime task is to provide care for their patients, there is a general trend away from the concept of the importance of the individual patient to caring for populations. Whether we

---

Exercise 12.1 To identify the building blocks for providing
optimum quality care

1. Is there a clear direction or strategic plan for the practice?

2. Is there commitment by the senior members of the practice to the strategic plan?

3. Has the strategic plan been shared with the members of the practice team?

4. Do all members of the practice team have a clear idea of the tasks for the practice and the priorities?

5. Are there adequate systems in place to achieve the tasks?

6. Has there been adequate training to achieve the tasks?

7. Does the practice have systems for giving feedback, both formal and informal?

---

are aiming for excellence in the individual consultation or excellence in providing preventative services, general practitioners are dependent on efficient management to allow them to provide that care. During the training year there is considerable focus on the interaction between the doctor and the patient. Registrars are strongly encouraged to record and review their consulting styles, yet if the appointments system is inadequate or there is no mechanism for recording visit requests, patient care will be compromised. Good management is related to having good systems for practice administration. There also needs to be clear direction, which is based on opinion gathered from the grass roots, and formulated into a plan which is shared effectively with everyone concerned. It may be useful to consider your own practice organization using Exercise 12.1.

Developing a strategic plan for a practice is an essential part of improving quality of care. Ideally the partners and the practice manager, with perhaps the practice nurse, will define the practice strategy. All too often practices are unwilling to set aside time for this important task. This makes implementation difficult but not impossible. There are many practices where one person takes a leadership role, having a clear vision of the future and taking the practice or the profession forward.

If the strategic plan has been developed by all the partners there should be commitment to it. If the plan is unwritten but agreed over time there can still be strong commitment. If there is no written document it may be difficult but not impossible to share the direction of the practice with other team members. A clear written document helps each member of the team to understand how their individual role fits into the practice development.

Exercise 12.2 sets out one way of developing a strategic plan. The important part of the exercise is reaching a common vision; where all members of the practice team are working towards a common goal the practice is likely to be efficient and content. Reaching agreement on the common goal can be difficult; often it needs delicate modification of words. This part of the strategic plan is so important that a practice might consider bringing in an expert facilitator, who will be familiar with working in groups, and who is likely to be aware when members of the group are irritated. Sometimes a practice working alone will become so enthusiastic about their future that they will fail to recognize if one member of the group is expressing verbally or non-verbally that they are not in agreement. To miss these vital clues could be detrimental to ownership and implementation of the plan.

Before we can hope to provide excellent clinical care for our patients, our internal practice systems are likely to need overhauling. General practice has grown considerably in the last ten years. Our support staff have multiplied and they have each become more highly skilled in their work. Ten years ago one of the senior receptionists might have doubled up as the administrator, and the other receptionists may have worked on the computer when they were required or had the time. Now we usually have a member of the team who has extensive computer skills and a practice manager who is responsible for the day to day running of the practice. When considering how a practice needs to improve it is important to remember that although we are all working towards providing care for our patients, we are more effective in that task if our internal mechanisms are efficient.

When things go wrong it is easy to blame a member of staff, but if you reflect on the errors in your own practice you will soon realize that most are caused by inadequate systems rather than people. Exercise 12.3 illustrates how we are dependent on a number of different people within the practice team. Unless each member of the team understands how their individual task is important to the smooth running of the practice they are likely not to see the importance of adhering to expected standards.

EVALUATING QUALITY—AUDIT

Once a practice has defined the sort of care it wants to provide and the management systems that will be needed to deliver that care, then it can begin to audit its work and make changes to achieve that goal. Audit is the systematic measuring of local attainment of standards against peer standards. If all members of the practice team are involved in defining the sort of care which the practice should provide they are likely to want to be involved in trying to establish if it is being achieved. They are likely to collect information for audit willingly and accurately.

It may be difficult for a young doctor to involve the whole practice in audit

Exercise 12.2 To develop a strategic plan (adapted from Pendleton, King)

Preparation for a strategic planning day

The practice will need to decide who is to attend the day and set a date where everyone concerned will attend. If a facilitator is to be used this will need arranging and the facilitator will need briefing. If not all members of the practice team are going to attend there will need to be explanation as to what is likely to occur and there should be an opportunity for each member of the team to make their views known. Who attends the day will be a matter for each practice to decide. Six to eight people is a good size for a group. All the partners will need to be present. A suitable venue needs to be chosen and arrangements made for the clinical care of patients.

Stage 1. Setting the vision

1. Each person should imagine that it is five years in the future and that the practice has been given an award for merit in five areas.

2. Each person should take about thirty minutes to write down the areas which he or she would like to be awarded a merit for excellent performance.

An example might be: *The practice will provide excellent clinical care for the registered patients.*

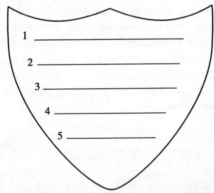

3. Each person should take about ten minutes to present their vision of the practice to the rest of the group. The exercise is helped if each person can write his five vision statements on a large sheet of paper.

4. The group should consider each vision in turn and try to draw together a collective vision.

5. At the end of stage 1 the group should have five statements describing the sort of practice they would like to be.

To develop a strategic plan (*continued*)

Stage 2. Where are we now?

1. Working together the group members should describe the current state in the practice for each of the five statements.

Stage 3. Identifying helping and hindering forces

1. For each of the statements the group should identify the factors which will help them reach their vision and the factors which will hinder them reaching their vision.

Helping factors	Hindering factors
1.	
2.	
3.	
4.	
5.	
6.	

Stage 4. Developing a plan

1. The group should now identify a plan which will reduce the hindering forces and enhance the helping forces. If time is limited, concentrating on reducing the hindering forces will be more effective.

2. The plan should be:

Specific	What exactly should we do?
Measurable	How will we know when we have reached our goal?
Achievable	Are we being realistic?
Relevant	Is it important now?
Trackable	How will we monitor progress?

3. At the end of the exercise the practice should have a list of tasks which need to be completed by defined dates. Each task should have the name of a member of the practice attached to it. That person will take responsibility for ensuring that the task is completed.

4. One person should be responsible for writing up the plan.

Exercise 12.3 To identify internal practice consumers and the level of service provided

1. Each member of the practice should take ten minutes to identify all the other members of the practice team for whom she/he provides a service.

2. For each member she/he has identified she/he should define what she/he provides and what standard she/he believes she/he is providing.

   Example: The practice filing clerk provides a service to:

   The receptionist—she makes sure that the records are placed in the correct slot on the shelf.
   The doctor—she makes sure that all correspondence relating to the patient is filed in the correct order in the medical records.
   The practice manager—she makes sure that when records are returned to the shelf that no signed FP1001 forms are left in the records.
   The audit clerk—records are extracted according to the protocol.

3. Each member of the practice team should then identify the other members of the practice who provide a service for them.

   Example: The practice filing clerk might expect:

   From the receptionist—to be given the surgery lists for extraction of the records in adequate time.
   From the doctor—notification when records are kept for dictation, etc., so that a tracer card can mark the shelves.
   From the practice manager—clear directions as to how tasks are to be carried out and what freedom for modification she has.
   From the audit clerk—information about any audits, particularly those that relate to her work.

---

soon after becoming a partner, however that should not deter them from continuing the ethic gained during their training practice of looking critically at their own work. Audit is not a difficult exercise. It is not research, although it may generate questions which lead to research, and it is more than just counting. Audit is about setting standards, seeing if you attain them, changing your behaviour if you don't, and checking again to make sure you have attained them the second time. A guide to undertaking audit is included in the final section of this book.

Significant event analysis should identify what goes well or badly and why, so that the practice can learn and encourage the good whilst minimizing the undesirable:

The Village practice was proud of the care it provided for its patients; they were upset when the practice manager received a letter from Mrs Phillips complaining about the delay in visiting her. The partners remembered the day well, the senior partner had been away and the junior partner's wife had gone into premature labour, leaving two doctors working.

The practice decided that they should set time aside with all the people concerned, including doctors, manager, receptionist, and midwife. Dr Brown spoke first. He had looked after the lady until his annual leave, he had visited over the week-end when she had complained about soreness in her breasts, he had not thought to mention it to the other partners as she was still being visited by the midwife. The midwife spoke next. She had seen Mrs Phillips on the day concerned, she had told her that a doctor would call later that morning. As the doctors were busy, she had asked the receptionist to put Mrs Phillips' name in the visit book. The receptionist said that she had done as requested and put the medical records in the visit box. As Dr Brown was away she had not indicated which doctor was to visit. She had also taken a telephone message from Mrs Phillips during the afternoon. She had reassured her that the doctors were still doing their visits and would be round shortly.

Dr Smith had been the duty doctor that day: it had been particularly busy, she had been telephoned by Mrs Phillips in the evening asking why no doctor had visited. She had gone straight out to find a lady with a breast abscess whom she had admitted for drainage. She had apologized for the delay, explaining that they had been very busy. When she looked in the visit book she had found that she had put her initials by Mrs Phillips' name but the current layout of the book made it difficult to be clear that she had taken the visit. As the records were arranged for routine maternity visiting it had not caught her eye from the visit box.

The practice agreed that arrangements for taking visits needed to be clearer. They agreed that the visit book should be set out to allow reception staff to record the date and time of the visit request, there should be a column for them to tick when they had put out the records and a column for the doctor's initials. The partners agreed that they should try to minimize the number of times that two doctors were absent at one time. The practice manager wrote to Mrs Phillips expressing the practice's concern about the delay and letting her know that the practice had made changes to prevent similar events.

Significant event analysis allows a practice to get together in a non-threatening way to go through events leading up to a problem or a success. It should be held in a non-threatening format with all members of the team involved in the event contributing to the discussion.

SUMMARY

All general practitioners like to be proud of the care that they provide. We all need constant feedback to help us develop our clinical skills. However, many of us forget the contribution of other members of the practice team to good quality care. Many receptionists are far more meticulous than general practitioners when completing paperwork, either for audit or for managing patient populations. We should not be frightened to allow them to develop their skills, leaving us free to do what we do best, look after patients. The most important aspect of delivering good quality care is for the practice to be clear how it wants to develop, for all members of the practice team to understand that plan, and to work within it to develop and evaluate their own skills.

REFERENCES

1. Pendleton, D., Schofield, T., Havelock, P., and Tate, P. *The consultation: an approach to learning and teaching.* Oxford: Oxford University Press, 1984.
2. What Sort of Doctor Working Party. *What sort of doctor?* Report from general practice 23. London: Royal College of General Practitioners, 1985.

Part 3

Getting it right

13 Clinical care and clinical audit

INTRODUCTION

General practitioners are, first and foremost, clinicians. An average full time general practitioner will undertake over 7500 consultations per year, the content of which varies from a minor cough to an acute myocardial infarction.[1] This is not, however, a textbook of clinical medicine and it would be invidious to attempt to sketch good clinical care for individual conditions. However, there are principles which underpin our clinical behaviour which we need to consider, and these are the subject of this chapter.

EVIDENCE BASED MEDICINE

Although the term 'evidence based medicine' has recently gained common currency[2,3] the concept has been with us since medicine became a science. The purpose of most medical research is to provide evidence which is either directly or indirectly of value to clinicians in delivering patient care. The novelty in the current vogue for evidence based medicine is the concept that we must learn to access and apply existing knowledge more effectively, and we must identify those areas of our practice for which there is no evidence and encourage research.

The NHS research and development strategy[4] is based on the latter imperative—in each research area, a group of people with special interest meet to define the major (in resource or clinical care respects) unanswered questions; these are then circulated to the research community and research bids are called for; and research is then commissioned which meets the needs of the health service rather than the whims of researchers.[5] As this programme is delivered, and it will take between three and five years before its effects can be assessed, we should see an increase in evidence of direct relevance to our clinical lives.

However, the first part of the challenge in evidence based medicine impinges more immediately on our work as general practitioners. The diffusion of 'facts' from research hypotheses to changes in clinical practice is an opaque process called dissemination. In industry it is called innovation and an 'S' shaped curve is described. In the first, slow phase the innovators—those that like to be seen to be ahead of the pack, the risk takers—try an idea and either gain a competitive advantage or find that the new idea doesn't work. If the innovators are seen to be successful, the majority then quickly adopt the idea, leaving a small group of laggards to slowly adopt the idea over time.

In general practice this was seen graphically with the advent of computerization (see Chapter 1). It took 20 years from the late 1960s for the innovators to convince the majority that the benefits of computers outweighed the disadvantages—especially the cost. However, in the next five years over 70 per cent of practices computerized leaving, now, only one in ten as the late adopters. Some of these will never computerize—there are still farms which only use shire horses—and as they find themselves increasingly marginalized in the health service they may survive by making a virtue of their 'old fashioned care'.

This model for the diffusion of innovation holds good for individual drugs except that there is a rebound phenomenon. New products raise expectations as the innovators often over-sell the benefits. Early trials are often conducted on highly selected groups and comparisons are made to placebo rather than existing drugs; colleagues who are the first to use the drug trumpet the benefits while conveniently ignoring non-responders or side-effects. As the drug is adopted by the majority a more cynical view begins to prevail. This might lead to a drug's withdrawal, as in the Opren case, but more usually it leads to an over-pessimistic view of the drug's effectiveness. Eventually, through a series of oscillations, the drug finds its rightful place in our formularies and an understanding is reached concerning the balance of effects and side-effects, and the patients most likely to benefit.

As Fig. 13.1 shows, the expert reviewers took over a decade before they were

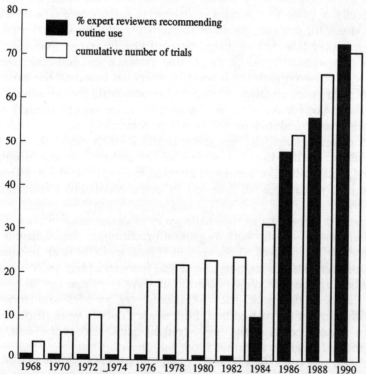

Fig. 13.1. Thrombolytic therapy for acute heart attack: the delay between proving success of therapy and this advice appearing in most medical reviews.[6]

prepared to recommend a treatment which the literature had shown to be effective.[6] After the expert reviewers support thrombolysis, there is a further lag before clinical practice catches up; even now many patients with acute myocardial infarction do not receive thrombolysis.[7] The use of aspirin in acute myocardial infarction offers a further, slightly different illustration. Clinical trials[8] purported to show that starting aspirin early after an acute myocardial infarction reduced deaths by about a fifth, and this was disseminated as advice for all patients without a specific contraindication who had a suspected myocardial infarction to be given 150 mg of aspirin as soon as possible—by a relative, general practitioner, or ambulance man, but certainly before hospital admission.[7,9] As this policy was made known throughout the country, it became clear that the original evidence related to the effect of a four week course of aspirin started soon, but not immediately, after the myocardial infarction, and that there was no evidence for the effectiveness of a single dose at the time of infarction.[10] There will now, no doubt, be a revision of the proclaimed policy and a more accurate one will be drafted; the late adopters will either go straight to the new policy or will erroneously adopt the old policy before finally arriving at the new.

This should not be taken as concrete evidence for therapeutic conservatism. Each doctor will be an innovator for some ideas, and a late adopter of others. But there are responsibilities on the innovators. They should innovate knowingly, being prepared to recant if the innovation is not successful; and they must critically evaluate the effectiveness of the innovation. In a perfect world, good ideas will be quickly shown to be beneficial and that information will be widely and authoritatively known as soon as possible—with the dissemination of adverse comment on poor innovations occurring just as effectively. Lastly, innovators must, of course, be very careful to ensure that all innovations are ethical and, at least theoretically, justifiable. This stricture applies to new procedures just as much as it does to new drugs.[11]

We are usually, however, in the majority group that adopts new ideas after the innovators have had their say. How can we sort the wheat from the chaff? How can we keep up-to-date, and avoid joining the Luddites in the late adopting group? This has always presented considerable problems for general practitioners whose breadth of knowledge is greater than in any other discipline.

General practitioners often defer to 'experts'. Lectures delivered by consultants are still a popular mode of continuing medical education, and general practitioner prescribing is often fundamentally influenced by the prescribing patterns of hospital colleagues in out-patients. While this method of diffusion has its merits, it also has limitations. Many lectures concern cases that general practitioners do not see; dermatologists tend to show slides of florid pemphigoid rather than mild psoriasis. And consultants are often early adopters of new drugs in their areas of special interest, only to abandon them with equal alacrity.

Obviously, a general practitioner in a perfect world would be reading and critically evaluating all the literature concerning each innovation before adopting it. This would, however, be quite unrealistic. The early trials of drugs are published in inaccessible pharmacological journals, often in foreign languages.

Even if the literature was fully available, the time taken to undertake a full review in just one area—say, for one drug—would be formidable, and much evidence would conflict. Lastly, some of the studies will purport to demonstrate that an innovation is ineffective, when this is solely an artifact of the 'power' (the capacity of the numbers of cases involved in the study to show a significant difference) of the study. This latter problem is overcome by pooling studies to increase their collective power in a process called meta-analysis.[12-15] Rather than get swamped, a good general practitioner will adopt a selective strategy towards innovation. The following is a selective strategy for keeping up-to-date:

1. Listen to, but do not slavishly imitate, partners, other general practitioners, and hospital colleagues.

2. Read the abstracts of the research literature in at least two peer review journals such as the British Medical Journal, British Journal of General Practice, The Lancet, Family Practice, or the European Journal of General Practice. Particularly concentrate on research from or about general practice and general medicine.

3. Read and keep copies of editorials or review articles which cover general practice topics.

4. Attend continuing medical education events in areas that cause you doubt and concern, preparing first by re-reading articles kept in (3).

5. Ensure that there is support from at least two of the four above sources before deciding on a significant change in clinical practice.

Clearly any general practitioner who wishes to keep up-to-date needs to be selective on two levels—selective concerning what they read and selective concerning what weight they give each item of evidence. An important skill involves, therefore, the assessment of the significance of any article, especially an original research article. There are a few key questions that need to be addressed:

1. Does this study pose a question of relevance to my work?

We usually select interesting articles on the basis of their titles. However, after being enticed into the abstract, we often discover that the main question is not relevant to our clinical lives. The title might suggest that an article concerned the effect of occupation on consulting rates; on reading the study aims in the abstract it becomes clear that the occupational groups are different grades of workers in an Hungarian tractor factory, and the consultations are with an occupational health service. Suddenly the urge to turn the page becomes uncontrollable.

2. Are the results of relevance to my work?

We are all, as general practitioners, concerned to offer high quality care for our patients with diabetes. If research examined the benefits of an insulin pump which adjusted the insulin dose according to the blood sugar, we would all be interested; however, we would want to know whether the equipment was practical, available, affordable, and reliable. If the trial involved patients being attached to a non-ambulant machine, we might be interested at a theoretical level but would realize that this work was not immediately of applicability to our patients. Equally, some articles sound irrelevant but contain something of relevance and interest; these are the ones that colleagues quote and that you rush off to check up on.

3. If true, would the findings alter my practice?

Much published research serves only to reinforce our prejudices and established clinical behaviour. These are valuable both in bolstering our current practice and in acting as a counter-weight to an article which proclaims the opposite. However, when a finding surprises us we need to pause and evaluate its implications. Only if we believe that this finding has a potential to alter our behaviour, need we continue our critical appraisal of the article.

4. Can the results be relied on?

There are numerous ways in which a piece of research can mislead the reader:

a. The experimental design is inappropriate. This is a complex area which deserves extensive discussion beyond the scope of this book, but there are some general principles to watch out for. A study may simply describe the reality as it exists (for example, the number of general practitioners who carry a peak flow meter as part of their emergency kit). For these studies you need to be sure that the sample was representative (how did they decide who to ask?), the response rate was sufficient, and that opinion is not mixed with fact. To pursue this latter point, lots of studies tell us what people think that they do (and more likely what they think they ought to do) but that is not the same as telling us what they really do. Many descriptive studies use qualitative methods—they seek rich data in depth to increase understanding, rather than superficial data in breadth to prove association—which need to be applied rigorously if they are to be relied on; for these you need to build up a knowledge of accepted methodologies and look for the track record of the authors before relying too heavily on their findings.

Many studies report the effects of interventions. The holy grail of these studies is the randomized control trial but these are difficult to undertake in general practice—it is truly hard to randomize half your patients to receive, say, physiotherapy while preventing the other half from getting the service. Often the researchers report the situation before the intervention and compare it to the situation afterwards, perhaps comparing the findings to a control site where no intervention occurred. Less satisfactory is a comparison between two groups at one point in time, one group having experienced one particular type of care; this, however, is unavoidable if you wanted, for example, to see if different patient list sizes influenced night visit rates.

Sometimes the data are collected retrospectively, but it is usually more rigorous if the data are recorded prospectively. The critical reader needs to reflect on the research question and then consider the research method used; only if the design was the most appropriate for the circumstances should the findings pass this test.

b. The power of the study is too low. By this it is meant that the sample size was too small to stand a reasonable chance of demonstrating a meaningful difference; thus a negative finding cannot be relied on. We might all regard a five per cent reduction in night visits as worth achieving providing the cost was not excessive; the numbers of night visits in a single practice in one year would not be sufficient to demonstrate a significant ($p < 0.05$—see below) difference between chance events and a new system for out-of-hours care which achieved just such a reduction. To reach statistical significance, a larger sample would be required.

c. The power of the study is too large. If, however, hundreds of practices were enrolled in the new system for out-of-hours care there might be a statistically significant difference shown when the change was only a drop of one per cent in night visits. While reaching significance, and thus pleasing editors and statisticians, you need to ask if the difference shown was worth achieving clinically or managerially.

d. The author's conclusions exceed the evidence. Every researcher feels a temptation to proclaim research findings from the roof-top. Having slaved over hot data for months, there is a natural desire to emphasize the great importance of the results. A good article, however, openly admits to the limitations inherent in the study design, is cautious about findings which conflict with the existing literature, and takes a realistic approach to interpreting their importance. The river of knowledge is built up incrementally from the droplets of thousands of research articles, and none makes such a splash that it overwhelms the others. Lastly, do please remember what a 'p' value tells us—'$p = 0.05$' says that this finding would be expected to happen by chance only one time in twenty; '$p = 0.01$' is once in a hundred: they do not say 'this finding is totally true and can be relied on'. Obviously, the smaller the value of p, the less likely is the finding to be a chance finding. But a study that looks for associations between fifty variables will have 1225 pairs of comparisons, and over 60 significant ($p < 0.05$) findings might be expected by chance; so look for authors that set themselves rigorous levels of evidence.

e. Do I have faith in this research team? This is the indefinable element in the critical appraisal of an article. We are much more likely to accept a finding from a research team with a track record in the area and who has offered us reliable findings in the past. We trust the clinical opinion of some colleagues more than others and it is also true of research. This is not to say that you should disregard findings from unknown (to you) researchers; but naturally we put more weight on the findings of those we respect.

5. What else do I need to know before I act?

Often a research paper only addresses a very limited question. A study might show that one anti-depressant achieves a faster resolution of symptoms of depression than another. Next you need to consider side-effects, costs, availability, and the opinion of local psychiatrists. Seldom can a single research paper on its own guide you to a definitive decision concerning clinical or managerial behaviour.

ACCESSING THE EVIDENCE

For many general practitioners, evidence is gained opportunistically. Whatever happens to be in their journals and whatever happens to be the subjects of local postgraduate education forms the basis of their evidence. All have access to some books and many have reasonably comprehensive libraries, so systematic enquiry can, and does, occur. In the next few years, however, physical barriers to accessing the evidence will be lifted. With the arrival of electronic links into databases—such as the BMA's link into Medline—general practitioners, wherever they are, will be able to undertake a literature search. As the Internet becomes more established, the major journals will be available, as the British Medical Journal is already, and a 'library' of back numbers will accumulate. Lastly, sources of more static and reference information are increasingly available both through networks and on CD-ROM.

Let us speculate that a general practitioner of the future wishes to review the practice's care of patients dying at home. She will consult the current definitive texts on screen, and will call up all the guidelines and protocols (see below) written for palliative and terminal care. A search of the recent literature will yield a list of, say, fifty relevant articles of which she chooses five to read in detail; these are summoned electronically. After the practice has digested the evidence, discussed its proposals within the team and with colleagues in the local hospice, a protocol is agreed and circulated. That protocol, with references to the literature that supports it, is then entered on the network for others to consult. Since this file will include the practice's network address, other general practitioners will comment on and question aspects of the practice protocol, helping the original practice when it reviews its protocol, standards, and criteria. These regular updates appear on the network and, in time, include the results of the practice audits of palliative care.

In the meantime, a young general practitioner will be working towards a fluency with the literature of the discipline, building up a library of books, journals, and cuttings, and learning how to use electronic communications. All the access in the world will not, of course, improve patient care unless the physician between the two has a commitment to evidence based medicine, and that commitment needs nurturing.

GUIDELINES AND PROTOCOLS

It seems obvious that the easiest way to interpret the plethora of evidence into practical suggestions for clinical care is to convene a group of experts, equip them with all the literature, time, and secretarial support, and ask them to write the guidelines for the rest of us to use.[16,17] While this approach has merits, it also has considerable disadvantages.[18]

Often the 'evidence' is incomplete or contradictory. This leads the experts to make statements which are more subjective than objective—based more on current 'best practice' than on evaluation. If there is good evidence in some areas of care for a problem, such as the use of inhaler steroids in asthma, there may be little evidence for, say, the frequency of review. The experts are confronted with a difficult choice: either they produce guidelines which ignore major aspects of the delivery of care because the evidence is lacking, or they are comprehensive but stray beyond the evidence. In the early days they usually chose the latter course.

All too often the 'experts' are predominantly from a group that differs significantly from those for whom the guidelines are recommended—in carica-ture a group of consultants with a token general practitioner deciding what care should be delivered by primary care teams. Further, much of their evidence is derived from highly selected groups of patients treated in the hospital setting and there may be substantial doubts concerning the transferability of the findings.[19]

The alternative scenario, however, might be thought to be quite unrealistic—all practices reinventing the wheel for every condition. There is, fortunately, a middle road. We should be identifying and using guidelines which have these characteristics:

1. The guideline has been written by a group which is predominantly drawn from the group to which it is targeted: guidelines for general practice by general practitioners and practice nurses, with patients, consultants, and others to assist.

2. Every criterion which is derived from the literature is clearly referenced with a brief supporting explanation.

3. Every statement or criterion which is not supported by evidence should be clearly labelled as a 'recommended best practice'.

4. The guideline should be explicit concerning the patient group that it ad-dresses (not just patients with asthma but, say, adults with mild or moderate asthma) and to whom it is targeted.

5. Every guideline should be accompanied by evidence of piloting where there are substantial differences between recommended practice and existing clinical care.

The authors know of no guidelines which currently meet these strictures; this illustrates the credibility problem that surrounds guideline development.

So, what exactly is a guideline? A guideline concerns itself with general statements concerning a particular condition in a defined group of patients, as for example those by the World Health Organization and the International

Society of Hypertension guidelines for the management of mild hypertension,[16] those for asthma,[17] or those on the diagnosis and treatment of non-insulin dependent diabetes from the British Thoracic Society and two Royal Colleges.[20]

A practice needs to be aware of local, national, and international guidelines when deciding what it is to offer as care. Sometimes it will aspire to higher levels of care than described in a guideline; sometimes local circumstances dictate lower standards. However, the important concept is that deviations from the accepted norms of good care should be explicit and justifiable.

Having considered the available guidelines and research evidence, a practice will then discuss what it wishes to sign up to—this is a protocol. A protocol does not have to be a lengthy document, but what evidence there is to support it should be available. A protocol covers the target population, the method of identification of cases including diagnostic criteria, action at first consultation, frequency and content of review, and management options and objectives. It will then state a number of criteria (statements of care to be achieved) and standards (the extent to which they will be achieved). As an example, one practice's protocol for hypothyroidism is reproduced on page 146.

CLINICAL AUDIT

Protocols such as the example reproduced here, with criteria and standards, are the basis for clinical audit.

Table 13.1 shows how one practice matched up to its criteria. This practice decided to rely on the computer entries for auditing its standards, which can distort the results—in 1993 very few blood results were being entered onto the computer. However, this audit takes no time to execute and, especially if done regularly with inter-doctor comparisons, it can help a practice to improve its clinical care.

This protocol approach has significant limitations. It cannot be applied to many areas of primary care where there is no evidence concerning appropriate care; it must never be seen as 'cookbook medicine' which negates the responsibility of all clinicians to exercise judgement; and most importantly it must never become a tool to punish patients. To pursue this latter point, we have a clear responsibility to make high quality of care available and accessible to all appropriate patients, and to ensure that patients are aware of the importance of availing themselves of that care. We may even have a responsibility to gently pursue non-attenders through reminders. But we must respect patient autonomy and the right for people to choose whether or not, within limits, to accept medical advice. That is why the practice in the example protocol has set a standard of 80 per cent for recording of thyroid function test results and weight within the previous 14 months. Some patients will default and that is a reality of patient care—they will, however, be opportunistically checked when they attend for some other problem.

However, such audits—based on evidence which has been codified into a guidelines, a protocol, and then criteria and standards—can be undertaken in

An example protocol for hypothyroidism

Target Group:	All patients diagnosed as having hypothroidism
	At risk patients: I^{131} therapy
	Thyroid surgery
	Lithium therapy
	Adult Down's syndrome
	Insulin dependent diabetes
	Pernicious anaemia
	Addison's disease
	Dementia
Diagnostic criteria:	Raised TSH
First consultation:	Clinical, menstrual, family and drug histories
	Examination: Features
	Extremities
	CVS–BP, pulse rate, HS, apex
	Lungs
	Reflexes
	Weight
	TFTs, FBC, ESR
	Autoimmune antibodies
	Consider ECG, CXR
Review interval	At least annually
Review content:	At risk patients: Annual TSH
	If hypothyroid: Clinical history
	Pulse
	Weight
	Annual TSH
Management:	Thyroxine (gradual introduction, especially in IHD)
Clinical objective:	TSH in normal range

CRITERIA	STANDARDS
At risk patients having TSH within 18 months	To be achieved 80%
Hypothyroid patients diagnosed in the past 10 years to have a raised TSH prior to treatment	To be achieved 95%
Hypothyroid patients to have TSH within 14 months	To be achieved 80%
Hypothyroid patients to have BMI within 14 months	To be achieved 80%
Hypothyroid patients to have last TSH in normal range	To be achieved 80%

many areas of our care with benefit. One of the authors' practice undertake regular audits against protocols for asthma, diabetes, hyperlipidaemia, hypertension, hypothyroidism, smoking, alcohol consumption, weight and obesity, hormone replacement therapy, and contraception. Patients' charter areas—for

Table 13.1 Example of audit results for hypothyroidism

Criterion	Standard	Audit results		
		1993	1994	1995
Hypothyroid patients to have TSH recorded on computer within 14 months	80%	6%	55%	63%
Hypothyroid patients to have BMI recorded on computer within 14 months	80%	80%	90%	95%
Hypothyroid patients to have last TSH recorded on computer in normal range	80%	63%	63%	64%

example, appointment availability and duration of wait after appointment time—are highly amenable to audit.

Auditing process and outcomes

There is an important theoretical distinction between auditing process and auditing outcomes which tends to get blurred in practice. Avadis Donabedian coined the now famous triad of 'Structure, Process, and Outcome' as a conceptual framework for hospital auditing in the United States. At its simplest, the structures are numbers of beds and staff. The process covers numbers of admissions and lengths of stay, and outcomes include mortality, cure rates, and patient satisfaction. In many instances, however, there is no clear dividing line between structure and process, but the model has served us well. Its principal current function is to focus our thinking on outcomes.

Most general practitioners start 'auditing' by looking at prevalence and incidence—how many diabetic patients do we care for? This usually leads on to questions of the process of care—how often do we see our patients with hypertension and what do we do when we see them? Increasingly we are now asking: how much benefit do patients gain from the care we deliver? The traditional outcome measure, especially used in epidemiology, is death. It is easily recognized, routinely recorded, and has wide acceptance as a valid outcome measure for populations. It would not be suitable, self evidently, as an outcome measure for a practice's audit of minor surgery. The ideal characteristics of an outcome measure used in audit should be:

1. The outcome should occur with sufficient frequency in the audited population.

2. The outcome should vary with the quality of care. (This should either be supported by evidence from the literature—the most preferable—or by the consensus view of clinicians in the field.)

3. The outcome should be amenable to change in the short or medium term.

4. The outcome should reflect the value system of the clinicians, managers and, most importantly, patients. (There is little point in improving an outcome that nobody regards as important.)

5. Where the outcome measure used is a proxy for another outcome which is more difficult to measure, the proxy outcome should be as close to the desired outcome as possible.

6. The outcome should have a clear definition.

7. The outcome should be recorded in routine care and should be readily available from the practice computer.

Not all these criteria will be met by all outcome measures chosen, but where they are not met this should be explicitly understood. For example, an audit of asthma care may use a patient questionnaire (quality of life; severity and frequency of symptoms). This complies with every stricture except the need to use routinely collected data. The clinicians might also choose to audit the ratio of inhaled bronchodilators to steroids prescribed to these patients. Such a measure is open to two criticisms: it is a proxy for 'better control' but its interpretation is dependent on the severity of the patients audited (which is itself dependent on the alacrity of case finding), and it has little face validity as an outcome measure to most patients. The auditing of smoking among patients with asthma has more face validity, but might be criticized as being difficult to change and being too remote a proxy for asthma itself. Another outcome chosen for this audit might be the number of acute admissions for asthma. In a general population of asthmatics this will happen too rarely to comply with the first stricture, but this measure meets all the others and so may be valuable. Lastly, an audit could examine the ratio of the last recorded peak flow reading to the predicted peak flow. Here the doubt is raised as to the extent that such a measure reflects quality of care, and is associated with other outcomes. Peak flow readings at routine review are not necessarily a good indicator of overall control. Since few outcome measures meet all the criteria, you should look at a range of outcome measures, none perfect in themselves, but between them capable of building a picture of the quality of clinical care. There are three broad types of outcome measure:

1. Patient measures

Outcomes measures which examine the experience of patients must be a high priority. They may not, however, directly reflect the quality of care delivered—in some geographical areas patient compliance is easier to achieve than in others. Further, they may not be related to other outcomes—a patient may be very satisfied with a consultation in which they demand and are prescribed an inappropriate drug.

a. Patient satisfaction

Patient satisfaction with an episode of care—consultation, admission, etc.—or with an overall service is important but fraught. General questions often yield inappropriately high satisfaction ratings, whereas more detailed questioning demonstrates finer degrees of dissatisfaction. There are also concerns about the extent to which patient satisfaction accords with other outcome measures since 'satisfaction' requires a comparative judgement—if a patient is unaware of the potential care, then they may profess themselves highly satisfied with sub-standard care. Notwithstanding these issues, patient satisfaction surveys using validated instruments will continue to have a role to play in auditing outcomes.

b. Patient compliance

There is strong belief that patients respond to poor service by 'voting with their feet'. They do not attend appointments if they do not value the service being offered; they do not take a prescribed medicine if they are not persuaded of its advantages; they do not follow life-style advice if it is not given appropriately. Measures of patient compliance are very problematical since they may have only a tenuous connection to the quality of the care provided, but in some situations they are appropriate.

c. Patient life-style

Many life-style variables, such as body mass index, smoking, and alcohol, are now routinely recorded and can be used to reflect the overall preventive effect of a practice or other organization. As a repeat measure it can be of value, but the degree to which life-style variables can be changed by active intervention is doubtful. However, life-style measures have a popularity because they relate to a major priority (health promotion, as in the Government's Health of the Nation document) and are often easily audited.

2. Outcomes linked to specific events

Any episode of care, for example the fitting of an intra-uterine contraceptive device, can be audited by defining appropriate outcomes with appropriate time scales. Examples include the rate of infection, the number of coils that do not stay put, or the problems with subsequent periods.

3. Outcome measures in programmes of care

Much of our care is, however, delivered as part of a long-term programme of clinical care, designed to mitigate, avoid, or delay undesirable consequences. The care of patients with hypertension or asthma involves a long-term care programme where outcome measures linked to specific events in that programme are inappropriate. In many such patients we have clinical measures which are accepted as valid proxies for longer-term outcome. The maintenance of the TSH within the normal range (example, protocol above and Table 13.1) is considered an appropriate outcome proxy in myxoedema. In other situations, the clinical measure reflects only one aspect of care, as for example in the case of glycaemic control in diabetes. A patient with an excellent HbAlc might not consider themselves to have a good 'outcome' if they are registered blind with diabetic retinopathy. It is in programmes of care that clinical auditors must consider most carefully the possibility of using a range of outcomes, each of which might be limited as a single measure but which together build up a coherent picture of care.

Alternative methods for auditing outcomes

So far this chapter has emphasized the role of the clinical audit of groups of patients. Hospital clinicians have recognized for a long time the value of case based auditing. There is a strong tradition of using the post-mortem as an audit of clinical diagnosis, of confidential enquiries, and of case conferences such as perinatal morbidity meetings. There has been no such tradition in primary care. This has been largely due to the organization of practices and a predominance of care delivered by individuals rather than teams. These problems are now disappearing and a culture of critical appraisal of care is now becoming commonplace. As already mentioned in Chapters 5 and 12, this has made possible the introduction of significant event auditing.

Individual members of primary care teams undertaking significant event auditing record every event which they consider important on a sheet of paper. These events might be a myocardial infarction in a person under 70; an urgent visit to a patient with asthma; a new diagnosis of cancer; an attempted suicide; or a case of whooping cough. At a monthly meeting a selection of these cases are discussed in a constructive atmosphere which avoids blame allocation. The discussion is intended to help team members to increase their awareness of quality issues. Most significant events are outcomes of previous care. When a 51-year-old man has a myocardial infarction, the immediate care offered will be discussed. Was aspirin given? How long did the ambulance take to arrive? Did the doctor have the defibrillator and oxygen with him? But then the discussion will move on to the previous care recorded. Had his blood pressure been taken and if it was raised was anything done about it? Was his family history known? Was he a smoker and, if so, had he been offered advice and help to quit? Were there indications to do a cholesterol test and had one been done?

Such an approach carries the danger that individual outcomes disproportionately influence decisions about future care to others. Over-reaction to rare events is undesirable. It is, however, a method for overcoming the conundrum that important outcomes happen too rarely to be used as a measure of outcome in group audits. Most importantly, significant events auditing complements the psychological process of change, and change is required if improvements of care are to occur. Traditional group audits appeal to the intellect while significant event auditing appeals to the emotions—and change is an emotional process. Many doctors will justify a clinical belief by quoting a particular case and significant event auditing taps into this natural method for clinicians to evolve their standards of care.

Conversely, the danger of inappropriate decisions as a result of case discussions has to be recognized and a conventional audit is often required before a decision on changing clinical management is taken. The four results of a significant event audit are:

- celebration of high quality care delivered
- a conventional group audit
- immediate change on the basis of the discussion
- no action required.

APPLYING THE PRINCIPLES IN OTHER WAYS

Underpinning the development of protocols is the philosophy of accountability. We must make our clinical intentions explicit to ourselves, partners, the primary care team, patients, and those with whom we share care. The more explicit we are, the more we can hold ourselves and others to account. While there is no evidence that this places us at any increased legal risk—probably the reverse since protocol development can be seen as a defence against accusations of low standards—it does mean we are limiting our clinical freedom, if by that we mean our licence to behave illogically and inconsistently.

This limitation is best seen in cooperative working with colleagues to develop consistency of care. Many practices demonstrate this through the development of prescribing formularies. Some formulary decisions are clearly based on evidence of efficacy, effectiveness, absence of unwanted effects, and cost. Others are, however, pragmatic. The process of deriving a formulary can be highly educational in itself, can help partners to understand and learn from each other, and can help to create cohesion in the team.

The most important benefits of a formulary are, however, clinical. If a practice is using fewer drugs, understanding each better, and each partner is offering patients the same choices, then there is a much reduced scope for misunderstandings, interactions, and adverse effects. From a patient's perspective a formulary practice seems competent. Let us imagine how an asthmatic must view a practice where each partner prescribes a different brand of oral steroid in different initial dose and with a different regimen (reducing over a week, reducing over ten days, same dose for a week, same dose for ten days, etc.) in acute severe asthmatic attacks.

The habit of examining all aspects of the delivery of care, considering the evidence and guidelines, reaching local consensus, and auditing for compliance is the hallmark of a quality general practitioner and a quality general practice. It is a habit to nurture and develop despite the pressures and strains of working in the front line of the health service.

HEALTH-NEEDS ASSESSMENT

When a practice has defined the care that it expects to deliver to a particular groups of patients, it will develop a requirement to look at the care of its patients as a whole population. This allows the practice to identify strategic objectives and care needs that are not being met by the current services. Such a micro-epidemiological approach ('living epidemiology' in Professor Denis Periera Gray's concept, to distinguish it from the traditional epidemiological emphasis on mortality statistics) is the basis for commissioning of care to meet the overall needs of a practice.

There are four established methodologies for assessing the health-needs of a geographical area.[21] They each overlap and offer different insights into health problems. They are:

1. Use of health authority, census, and other population databases[21,22,23]
   For each of our practice areas there is a wealth of data to consult. Census results can be linked to postcode areas; life-style surveys are analysed by health district and locality; mortality data is available for small localities and so on. A visit to a member of the Department of Public Health in the health authority should be highly productive.

2. Use of practice derived information[21,24,25]
   We know a lot about our population if we consult our databases. We know about the prevalence of chronic diseases and the incidence of acute disease; we have detailed data on prescribing, investigations, and referrals; and we increasingly know about the life-style and life risks of our patients. And we have the results of all our clinical and managerial audits. If we can compare these data to other practices and the locality as a whole, it helps us to understand our population's health.

3. Rapid appraisal[21,26,27]
   Rapid appraisal is a new technique for gaining insight into the health-needs of a community through interviews with key informants. Although it sounds unscientific, it offers a valuable depth of insight that can help to prioritize information from other sources.

4. Patient surveys[21,28,29,30]
   Patients should have a say, and their views can help health professions to make more realistic decisions.

In time, health-needs assessment will be an integral part of every practice. It is a logical extension of the largely descriptive practice reports that many practices produce annually[31] and can draw together the protocols, clinical auditing, and routine data collection that are part of the life of a modern practice.

CONCLUSIONS

Guidelines, protocols, criteria, and standards are all aids to good clinical care. There is, however, no substitute for the caring doctor with high levels of inter-personal skills. However, such skills are themselves no substitute for good clinical care; the two elements of our discipline ('Cum Scientia Caritas' as the Royal College of General Practitioners' motto says) are complementary. We must be open to the evidence of science and the evidence of our emotions if we are to deliver the clinical care that our patients deserve.

REFERENCES

1. Royal College of General Practitioners, The Office of Population Censuses and Surveys, and the Department of Health. *Morbidity statistics from general practice, fourth national study* 1991–1992. London: OPCS, 1995.
2. Jones, R. and Kinmonth, A.-L. (ed.). *Evidence based medicine.* Oxford: Oxford University Press.
3. Ridsdale, L. *Evidence-based general practice.* London: Saunders, 1995.
4. NHS Management Executive. *NHS research and development strategy.* London: Department of Health, 1991.
5. Jones, R., Lamont, T., and Haines, A. Setting *priorities* for research and development in the NHS. *British Medical Journal,* 1995, in press.
6. Antman, E., Lau, J., Kupelnick, B., Mosteller, F., and Chalmers, T. A comparison of results of meta-analysis of randomised controlled trials and recommendations of clinical experts. *JAMA,* 1992; **268**: 240-8.
7. Reilly, R., Teasdale, S., McIlroy, S., and Pringle, M. *Audit of management of suspected heart attacks.* Lincoln: Lincolnshire Medical Audit Advisory Group, 1995.
8. Antiplatelet Trialists' collaboration. Collaborative overview of randomised controlled trials of antiplatelet therapy—I: Prevention of death, myocardial infarction, and stroke by prolonged antiplatelet therapy in various categories of patients. *British Medical Journal,* 1994; **308**: 81-106.
9. NHS Centre for Reviews and Dissemination (University of York). Aspirin and myocardial infarction. *Effectiveness Matters,* 1995, 1 (April).
10. Deeks, J., Watt, I., and Freemantle, N. Aspirin and acute myocardial infarction: clarifying the message. *British Journal of General Practice,* 1995; **45**: 395-6.
11. Haines, A. and Iliffe, S. Innovations in services and the appliance of science. *British Medical Journal,* 1995; **310**: 815-16.
12. Hazell, P., O'Connell, D., Heathcote, D., Robertson, J., and Henry, D. Efficacy of tricylic drugs in treating child and adolescent depression: a meta-analysis. *British Medical Journal,* 1995; **310**: 897-901.
13. Anderson, I. and Tomenson, B. Treatment discontinuation with selective serotonin reuptake inhibitors compared with tricyclic antidepressants: a meta-analysis. *British Medical Journal,* 1995; **310**: 1433-8.
14. Vander Strichele, R., Dezeure, E., and Bogaert, M. Systematic review of clinical efficacy of topical treatments for head lice. *British Medical Journal,* 1995; **311**: 604-8.
15. Eggar, M. and Davey-Smith, G. Misleading meta-analysis. *British Medical Journal,* 1995, **310**: 752-4.
16. World Health Organization/International Society of Hypertension, Milf Hypertension Liaison Committee. Summary of 1993 World Health Organisation/International Society of Hypertension guidelines for the management of mild hypertension. *British Medical Journal,* 1993, **307**: 1541-6.
17. British Thoracic Society, British Paediatric Association, Royal College of Physicians of London *et al.* Guidelines on the management of asthma. *Thorax,* 1993; **48**: Supplement S1-S24.

18. Royal College of General Practitioners. *The development and implementation of clinical guidelines*. London: RCGP, 1995.
19. Sweeney, K., Gray, D. P., Steele, R., and Evans, P. Use of warfarin in non-rheumatic atrial fibrillation: a commentary from general practice. *British Journal of General Practice*, 1995; **45**: 153-8.
20. British Diabetic Association, Research Unit of the Royal College of Physicians and the Royal College of General Practitioners. Guidelines for good practice in the diagnosis and treatment of non-insulin dependent diabetes mellitus. *Journal of the Royal College of Physicians of London*, 1993; **27**: 259-66.
21. Murray, S. and Graham, L. Practice based health needs assessment: use of four methods in a small neighbourhood. *British Medical Journal*, 1995; **310**: 1443-5.
22. Majeed, F., Cook, D., Poliniecki, J., and Martin, D. Using data from the 1991 census. *British Medical Journal*, 1995; **310**: 1511-4.
23. Majeed, F., Cook, D., Poliniecki, J., Griffiths, J., and Stones, C. Sociodemographic variables for general practices: use of census data. *British Medical Journal*, 1995; **310**: 1373-4.
24. Tennant, A., Fear, J., Pickering, A., Hillman, M., Cutts, A., and Chamberlain, M. Prevalence of knee problems in the population aged 55 years and over: identifying the need for knee arthroplasty. *British Medical Journal*, 1995; **310**: 1291-3.
25. Hopton, J. and Dlugolecka, M. Need and demand for primary health care: a comparative survey approach. *British Medical Journal*, 1995; **310**: 1369-73.
26. Hoskins, A., Saunders, P., and Forrest, J. A pilot study of a computerised assessment (AGE-PC) for the elderly in general practice. *Family Practice*, 1995; **12**: 28-31.
27. Shanks, J., Kheraj, S., and Fish, S. Better ways of assessing health needs in primary care. *British Medical Journal*, 1995; **310**: 480-1.
28. Hopton, J. and Dlugolecka, M. Patients' perceptions of need for primary health care services: useful for priority setting? *British Medical Journal*, 1995; **310**: 1237-40.
29. Lewis, J. and Williamson, V. Examining patient perceptions of quality care in general practice: comparison of quantitative and qualitative methods. *British Journal of General Practice*, 1995: **45**: 249-53.
30. Phip, I., McKee, K., Meldrum, P., Ballinger, B., Gilhooly, M., Gordon, S., Mutch, W., and Whittick, J. Community care for demented and non-demented elderly people: a comparison study of financial burden, service use, and unmet needs in family supporters. *British Medical Journal*, 1995; **310**: 1503-6.
31. Pringle, M. Practice Reports. In: *Medical audit and general practice* (2nd edn., ed., Marshall Marinker). London: BMJ Publishing Group, 1995.

14 Medical records

INTRODUCTION

Anyone who peruses medical records going back to 1948 (or before) can see how our use of the clinical record has changed. Many early entries, if legible, leave more to the imagination than we would now desire. Even if we allow for the (still) enormous variation in the standard of the contemporaneous medical record, it is now unusual to find notes where there is not an immunization card, a problem list, a health screening card, and so on. Furthermore, the *written* record is no longer unique. The argument about the electronic record has moved on from 'should we use the computer' to 'how much should we *not* put into the computer'. So we now have two systems, both of varying quality and content.

This chapter is concerned with medical records—their use, abuse, ownership, and development. It is not only concerned with factual issues but also with the values and beliefs embodied in the medical record. One of the great strengths of general medical practice has been said to be its diversity; no two doctors practice in the same way, just as no two patients present in the same way. Thus, 'doctors get the patients they deserve, and patients get the doctor they deserve.' At the same time, it has become apparent that this very diversity was also an obstacle to quality care. It is likely, therefore, that an incoming new partner will find that his or her experience is at variance with the local prevailing custom of the practice, no more so than in the arena of the medical records. Most of the record systems in the new practice will differ from those in the training practice, but they cannot all be changed at once! You need to be able to assess, review your options, prioritize, and then suggest change, if appropriate. Remember, however, that nobody has yet found the perfect records system for the rest of us.

HISTORICAL DEVELOPMENT

The medical record has changed. By and large, doctors don't change things unless for a good reason or unless change is imposed. In the case of medical records, change has occurred when they have ceased to function effectively and the expectations of the users—general practitioners and primary care teams— have changed. In 1948, the majority of medical practitioners were single handed. It was deemed unnecessary to make copious notes because no-one else would see them and general practitioners, with less administration and a simpler clinical agenda, could remember what happened anyway. Hence the minimalist entry to act as an aide memoire only. The locum, poor soul, just managed and no better. Litigation was unheard of, and GP's notes were not exposed in court.

After 1966 (see Chapter 1), general practitioners were encouraged to join in group partnership and a need arose for a note keeping system which allowed partners to have some idea of what had and was currently being done, or was planned. By 1980, a formal system of traineeship was in place which began to replace the assistantship schemes. Shortly afterwards, those who appointed vocational trainers saw the need for improvements in record keeping by training practices and they enforced good records by setting standards.

In addition, the job changed. The changes have been legion, and are described elsewhere in this book, but the principal recent changes have involved a much greater involvement with the management of chronic illness, and a shift from disease management to disease prevention. Both new areas called for a higher and more rigorous standard of note keeping, and also for recall systems. Although all practices adopted simple paper based systems initially, these are increasingly being replaced by electronic systems.

THE ELECTRONIC RECORD

In Chapter 1 the evolution of the computer record is described. Over 85 per cent of practices have now computerized, but the number of functions computerized and the content of the computer record varies. Every practice must decide its extent and pace of computerization, usually depending on the culture, organization, history, and finances of the practice. However, a new principal entering a practice needs to have a 'balance sheet' of pros and cons to refer to in discussions.

The use of the computer record to enhance the care of individual patients

A well written manual record can be a real help in a subsequent consultation. It can offer a description of the patient's problem, often using quotes direct from the patient; can include structured examination findings, including diagrams and subjective observations; may contain lists of alternative and speculative diagnoses; might record results of investigations; and, by virtue of the handwriting, identify the writer and even his or her mood at the time. We should discard this wealth of information at our peril. An electronic consultation record has to be superior to a manual record before it can be recommended, and yet a third of practices now say they have abandoned the paper consultation record in favour of a computer one. The evidence for their decision needs to be examined.

All major computer systems allow 'freetext'—text which is recorded and can be read, but cannot be analysed—and this should duplicate many of the features of the traditional record. Current computer systems cannot, however, record diagrams. The limitations of the current computer system lie in their coding structure. Read Codes, invented by Dr James Read and now maintained by the NHS Centre for Coding and Classification in Loughborough, offer a code for almost every conceivable diagnosis, procedure, and patient attribute. They do not, however, offer qualitative information. You cannot assign laterality (an inguinal hernia cannot be coded as left or right), severity, confidence of diagnosis (appendicitis is appendicitis, never ??appendicitis), or functional effects. These qualifiers are being created, but before they come, a total reliance on the computer consultation record seems premature. In practice visits to those using the 'paperless record,' it is often apparent that the computer record bears more of a resemblance to the manual record of 1945 than 1995: entries often contain shorthand, essential data is omitted because it is difficult to enter and a stranger consulting the record requires someone to act as interpreter.

Against these disadvantages must be placed the accessibility of the computer record—it can be entered from any connected terminal instantly, and can easily be transported out to patients' homes. The record can remind the doctor concerning activities which he or she should undertake for that patient through template or protocol screens, and can automatically warn of drug contraindications or interactions. Features of the record, such as past problems or smoking status, can be more easily available on the computer screen. Every general practitioner must weigh the pros and cons. However, a new principal is better occupied ensuring that the other aspects of the computer record are used effectively before trying to persuade reluctant partners to abandon the manual records entirely.

The use of computer records to enhance the care of groups of patients

It is in this area that clinical care can be most enhanced through computer use. Modern prevention programmes demand that patients are identified for call and recall, and that they are followed-up if they do not attend. Computerization has revolutionized our management of such programmes. By being able to identify patients with specific characteristics, a practice can ensure a quick and effective response to changing clinical knowledge. Recently, a practice decided that the evidence for active intervention with lipid lowering drugs was sufficiently compelling for those patients with proven arterial disease to warrant a change in practice policy. In place of benign neglect—repeated blood cholesterol estimations and encouragements to diet—the practice decided to recall all eligible patients for a blood fat estimation and to offer drug therapy. Eligible patients were easily identified from the computer problem entries, lists of patients were vetted by the doctors, and standard letters were generated.

The use of computer records for quality assurance

In Chapters 12 and 13, the central role of quality assurance has been explored. The possibility of auditing the care of groups of patients has been greatly enhanced through the use of computers. Clinical behaviour can be reinforced through templates and protocols linked to diagnoses—on reviewing a patient with diabetes the screen reminds the doctor of all the examinations that were agreed to constitute a review, including fundoscopy, foot pulses, and reflexes. The entries on the computer can be quickly analysed to show the level of recording (for example '79 per cent of hypertensives have a blood pressure recorded within the past 6 months') or, more usefully, the clinical control achieved (for example '72 per cent of the last recorded diastolic readings for patients with hypertension were beneath 90 mm Hg'). Comparisons to practice standards and criteria, to partners, and to other practices suddenly become possible. As discussed earlier, especially in Chapter 5, significant events auditing can be a powerful tool for quality assurance and computer problem entries can be used to assess lists of possible events for discussion.

The use of computers to save clinical time and effort

In the early days, computers were seen as an answer to the increasing bureaucracy of general practice. Staffing levels could be contained by using the computer to replace employees. As in many spheres of life, such efficiency savings have proved illusionary. It is possible to claim that computer repeat prescribing and call/recall systems save immense quantities of staff time, but non-computerized practices just do these tasks less efficiently.

The real gain in time has been through the great increase in managerial and informational sophistication that computers have allowed without requiring a proportionate increase in staff. The computers have, however, required some increases in staff. Many practices have data entry clerks and some have information officers who manage the computer system and the quality assurance of the practice.

One area where computers have enhanced functioning is in commissioning, which is quintessentially a process to improve overall patient care. It is inconceivable that a practice could hold a fund without computer support—indeed it is an entry requirement. But all practices are now commissioners of care in the primary care led NHS, and commissioning required health-needs assessment. As described in Chapter 12, a good health-needs assessment has many dimensions, but a vital one concerns the understanding of the health of the practice population as recorded on the practice computer.

Medico-legal implications

The medico-legal status of the computer record is confused. There has not yet been a test case in the courts in which a computer record was presented as evidence and its admissibility confirmed. It is likely, however, that a court would need to be confident of the originality of the record—that no retrospective tampering had occurred. This would require an audit trail which allows incorrect entries to be changed, but the original entry to be retained for later reading along with the date, time, and identity of the user when the original and the changed entry were generated. While confusion still reigns, caution in disbanding the manual record must again be recommended.

Further discussion on the role of technology in the practice setting occurs in Chapter 18. This review of the electronic patient record has been designed to equip a new principal with the issues and arguments which will be raised by moves towards a 'paperless' record.

THE CONTENT OF THE RECORD

The clinical and administrative record of a patient's care, whether manual or on a computer, contains a number of core elements. Firstly, it records the process of care. All consultations should be logged, including the identity of the person consulted and the mode/place of consultation (surgery, visit, telephone, third party, letter).

Whenever a patient sees a clinician, the record of that encounter must impart the key elements. In the Problem Orientated Medical Record (POMR) espoused by Lawrence Weed, the record should contain 'SOAP': Subjective, Objective, Assessment, Plan. A POMR entry is illustrated below; such structured entries can ensure that the record is meaningful to others and does not miss vital information. Problem orientated records are, of course, only an aid to good record keeping, and are not necessary for excellent communication.

The clinical record should contain all major or significant health events and diagnoses from a patient's past set out in a single list with dates of first presentation. It should contain dates and results, where appropriate, of all preventive procedures or record default. The latter includes those patients who positively state they do not wish to be considered for a procedure, such as cervical cytology. The medications historically prescribed to the patient should be clear from the record, including those currently being prescribed, with their dosage and compliance. Any drug reactions or allergies should be obvious. Dates and reasons for changes in medication should be discernable. All important historical investigation results should be available to the clinician, including ECGs and other graphic data. All referrals within and outside the practice should be easily discerned. External correspondence should be in date order and stored in a way that facilitates their reading. This is a tall order for a clinical record and it requires great effort and perseverance for a practice to maintain

---

An example of a problem orientated record entry

Date C S: Increasing lethargy over a week. Passing blood rectally for 'months'.
Probably lost weight. How much?

O: Looks anaemic. P–84 reg. BP 115/72 Abdomen—Liver palpable to 2 fingers PR—mass palpable in rectum: irregular and bled to touch

A: Rectal carcinoma with ?liver secondaries; Anaemia

P: Refer urgently to surgeon

exemplary records. The medium—manual or computer—is less important than the quality, organization, and presentation of the content.

WIDENING THE CLINICAL RECORD

Every practice has to decide on issues of access. There are cogent reasons for allowing all clinical members of the primary health care team access to read the clinical record, but that might not apply, for example, to a bath or school nurse, who has no legitimate requirement for routine access. Fundholding clerks often have a need to consult the clinical record to check on the progress of patients in secondary care and secretaries need to type letters. A wise practice facilitates access to the record for all those who need to use a particular record for a defined, legitimate primary care purpose, but is strict in condemning any access of a record for other purposes. In many practices, vicarious accessing of records is a sackable offence in the terms and conditions of employment, alongside deliberate breaches of confidentiality.

Who can write in the record is much more contentious still. There has been a natural prejudice against allowing the wider primary care team to write in the manual record simply because it risks an information explosion at the expense of clarity. Computer systems can, however, accommodate all team members making recordings and many practices encourage this.

A related but discrete issue for the medical records concerns litigation. The medico-legal status of computer records has already been alluded to; however, the problem is a general one applying to all medical records. A key function that they perform is to protect us and our team from litigation. Nobody keeps perfect records but we must all aspire to high quality medical records. Not only does clinical care demand it, as discussed earlier, but the courts and our patients expect it. However, the commonest cause of a failed defence by the insurance societies is poor records. An unwritten rule of good medical practice seems to be 'do what you want, but write it down'! And preferably so that someone can read it. Medical litigation is widely reported to be one of the doctor's greatest fears. A lost lawsuit damages you personally and harms morale in the whole practice. Each partner owes it to the others to ensure that the best defence is possible. This means that you should not just deliver good care, but be able to demonstrate from the written record that this was the case.

A last wider function of the medical record is for the preparation of reports. In addition to the contemporaneous record, reports for third parties rely heavily on correspondence. Ask ten GPs how they deal with the filing (or not!) of incoming letters and reports and you will, of course, get ten different replies. Again, a spectrum exists, from the defence society supported view that you throw nothing away, to the GP who bins the lot and writes a summarizing line in the notes. There is not a right or wrong way, of course. What works for you is fine, but, as with all the other processes we have looked at, we need to know what we do, why we do it, and whether we all do the same thing!

OWNERSHIP OF THE MEDICAL RECORD

The FP5 and FP6 state, at the bottom: 'property of the Secretary of State'. Hence, the Secretary of State (for Health) does not sell you continuation cards, but gives them to you, and thus retains ownership. The Secretary of State 'expects the GP to exercise due care in the preservation of the record and must take all steps to ensure that it is not lost or stolen.' However, since November 1991, that same Secretary of State is keen that we should exhibit them to the patients to which the records relate. So there are different sorts of ownership. Actual physical ownership belongs to the Department of Health. You are the owner of the comments included in the record, and the patient owns the right to see (part, at least) of the record. This all sounds very satisfactory, but what practical implications has it for our practices?

As you may have noticed, your computer's hard disk has no message from the Secretary of State. It belongs to you, the data within it belongs to you, but the patient has limited rights of access to that data. However, no one else has a right of access to it; after the patient has left your practice, either to someone else's practice or to go to that great partnership in the sky, the manual record must go with them. The computer record remains, however, with you.

The issues of physical ownership do not impinge substantially on the way in which we work. Although patients have the right to see parts of their medical record in law, very few have taken up the offer. Of greater interest to the systems we use is the question of moral ownership. Over the past few years, a trend has emerged towards sharing records with patients. Although there are still few doctors who 'trust' patients with their own records in toto, many have entrusted various aspects of the record to their patients. A practice should also be aware that the patient's record, building up over the years, is the only complete record of a patient's health and as such is a great asset to the clinician, clinical auditor, and researcher. Putting aside technicalities of ownership, the medical record which we retain is in our guardianship and we have a responsibility to care for and preserve it.

CONCLUSIONS

The medical record is the tool at the centre of our clinical lives. Whether manual, computerized or, more usually, both, it must be maintained as a key element of the communication between ourselves and colleagues within the practice, in secondary care, or with legitimate interests, such as doctors in insurance companies. The effort of maintaining quality records is rewarded in better patient care, greater job satisfaction with less stress, and improved practice management. But perhaps most importantly, good records offer peace of mind against confusion, mistakes, and litigation.

15 Practice organization and administration

DEVELOPMENT OF MANAGEMENT IN GENERAL PRACTICE

Throughout the earlier chapters reference has been made to the importance of organization and administration in the practice. A doctor may have the finest clinical skills and be an expert communicator but if his patients can never get to see him or if their consultations are constantly interrupted by the telephone or other members of the practice staff it is likely that he will not be an effective doctor. There has always been an element of management and organization in general practice—when general practitioners worked single handedly from their front room there was a need for them to organize their day and to have a system for recording house visits. Indeed before the inception of the NHS it was important that they had a system for ensuring that payment was made for their services.

As practices have grown, the need for effective organization has increased, and there has also mushroomed a plethora of books on the subject, some relating to medical management but others relating to management in general. One of the great strengths of general practice, and one of the important aspects of working in it, is the ability that we have to shape our own organization. If we choose we can take on an additional manager or receptionist, we may not receive additional funding, but we are not prevented from employing more staff. Probably the most significant event in relation to organization and administration in general practice was the 1966 charter. For the first time, general practitioners were not penalized for employing staff to help run the organization. Progressive practices used the opportunity to employ practice receptionists and possibly a part time practice nurse. During the next decade more practices took on staff to help with their organization. The forward thinking practices moved ahead, taking on a practice manager or training existing staff to take a managerial role. Towards the end of the 1980s practices were frustrated at their inability to employ a practice manager at a competitive rate. Although the 1990 contract was seen by some as an imposition and a loss of freedom, others saw it as an opportunity; they used the freedom created by fundholding and staff budgets to revamp their administrative structure.

A chapter on practice organization and administration may seem totally unnecessary if a young principal is working in a well run practice with an effective practice manager. Not everyone will be as fortunate and even if there is an effective manager in the practice in which you are working, circumstances may change. The chapter is divided into distinct areas, each of which could form a useful discussion for a young principals' group or for personal reflection. Throughout the chapter you may like to consider how your practice works in the area covered: could it be more efficient?

A 'WELL RUN' PRACTICE

A practice which is well organized may be a little like a person with good manners, they may be hard to define but it is obvious when they are not there. As with the other chapters, the use of exercises may help you to decide about the efficiency and effectiveness of your own practice organization. Just as it helps to break the consultation down into manageable sections to consider whether or not it is effective, it can be useful to consider a practice under five major headings: leadership, purposes, rewards, relationships, and structure. At the same time as the internal workings of a practice are considered, it is also essential to consider how it relates to the outside world. A practice may be very effective internally, but if it has no effective relationships with other organizations, such as the FSHA and secondary care, it will not be able to perform effectively.

Purposes

Earlier chapters have focused on developing a strategic plan. It may seem simplistic to ask what the purpose is for a general practice; of course it is to provide health care to the population. Individuals can vary in their understanding of what providing health care means; if two partners have different concepts of what the practice should be providing it can cause difficulties:

Dr Jones and Dr Smith were in partnership. Until 1990, they both had a similar view of their practice; they ran largely un-booked surgeries, responding to patient demand, they were both proud that their patients could see them without undue delay. When the MAAG formed, Dr Smith was invited to join; he soon learned about different ways of working, he introduced an appointment system and clinics for managing patients with asthma and diabetes, he began to audit the care the practice was providing. Dr Jones continued to run open surgeries, he began to feel resentful of Dr Smith's apparent decreased workload and he was irritated if patients complained about a delay in getting an appointment. It became apparent to the two partners that they had different aspirations for the practice and they decided to split.

In the chapter on managing change the importance of having a clear strategic plan was emphasized; without a clear plan often the purpose of the practice can get lost. Exercise 15.1 may help you think about the purpose of your practice.

Relationships

Relationships between members of the primary health care team and between the health care team and other bodies are fundamental. Stott[1] has described the importance of the core team, which includes people who work in the same building, and the extended team, which includes other individuals who have looser connections with the practice. Each practice team may be slightly different, what will be consistent is the need to develop the core team and to ensure effective relationships with the extended team. Beyond the extended team there

---

Exercise 15.1   To consider the purpose of the practice

These questions could be considered alone or in a practice meeting, alternatively they may be used in a young principals' group.

1. What is the main function of our practice?

2. How much agreement about our main function is there between the individuals working in the practice?

3. Are there clear, accepted objectives for the practice?

4. How well does our agreed main function fit with the rest of the NHS?

5. How well do we communicate our main function to others who work closely with us?

---

are other people with whom we work—the FHSA and secondary care are probably the most significant. Exercise 15.2 may help you consider relationships in your practice.

Rewards

When considering the rewards for working in your practice it is important to remember that rewards may be other than financial, and that different individuals seek different rewards. General practice is not one of the highest paid areas in which to work. Many of our staff, and indeed many doctors, work in the health service because they feel that it is a worthwhile job. They are prepared to take a lower income, knowing that they are seen as working in a respectable job.

Exercise 15.2   To consider relationships within the practice and with external organizations

1. How well do we work together?

2. Do we need to work together?

3. What produces conflict in our team?

4. How does the team deal with the conflict?

5. Does the conflict in the team disrupt our work?

6. How well do we support members of our team?

7. Does our practice enhance the self-esteem of the people working in it?

8. How is our practice seen by other groups that work with us?

Exercise 15.3   To consider the rewards for members of the health care team

1. What incentives do we have for people working in this practice?

2. Do members of our team know when they are working well?

3. Is good performance rewarded in our practice? If so, how?

4. Are there important tasks which need to be completed which seem to have no reward?

In dysfunctional organizations too much attention may be paid to higher order needs rather than taking care of basic needs. It is important that your staff have time to eat and rest, and perhaps most importantly to get to the toilet when they need. When these basic needs are catered for it is then possible to consider higher order needs such as self-fulfilment and personal growth. Exercise 15.3 poses some questions that might help you consider rewards in your practice.

Structure

Sometimes practices are limited by the building in which they work. If there is an opportunity to build new premises or modify existing ones it may be important to look at working arrangements and try to accommodate them. If it is not possible to change the fabric of the building it may be possible to move desks so that individuals with similar tasks or who inter-relate are working together. Team meetings are one structure that helps individuals consider a joint task. It may be worth reflecting on your building; minor modifications may alter working relationships.

Primary health care team meetings take place regularly across the country in most practices, but are they as effective as they might be? Teams meeting without an agenda, and without notes being taken, may be less useful then *ad hoc* meetings in a corridor. Could your practice work more effectively with less large team meetings which confine themselves to strategy and more task group meetings, solving particular issues?

The City Practice held a primary health care team meeting every week, mainly to discuss individual patients. The meetings seemed to drag on with little being achieved. The new practice manager felt uncomfortable in the meeting if patients were discussed as she was concerned about confidentiality. She also felt that the team should be discussing major policy issues, such as providing care for the increasing numbers of homeless in the locality. She proposed that the full team meet every two months with an agenda and a formal chairman, and that task groups should be set up to develop specific plans. In order to protect the interchange of information about patients she suggested that the partners allocate half an hour each day which could be used for individual team members to drop in, have a cup of coffee and discuss individual patients.

Leadership

Perhaps the most important aspect of any successful practice is effective leadership. Doctors often enter general practice because they had difficulty with the hierarchy of hospital life; they are understandably reluctant to recreate it in their practice. This may cause problems as without effective leadership the practice is likely to remain static. Leadership is not necessarily about driving forward all the time; Adair highlighted the importance of taking care of the task, the individual, and the team. If the balance between the three is uneven a leader may not be effective. The exercise to assess your management styles and your scores on the Belbin questionnaire may give you insight into your leadership style.

THE ROLE OF THE PRACTICE MANAGER

Having set out the building blocks for a successfully organized practice it is helpful to consider the part that a practice manager might play in practice organization. Each practice varies in the extent to which the practice manager or the partners organize the practice. At one extreme a partnership may be very hands on, delegating tasks to the practice manager, who in turn behaves more like a practice administrator. At the other extreme a partnership may allow a practice manager to take a full part in the practice, not just in the organization, and may reward them with a profit share of the business. Either model could result in an effective practice, but the former is not likely to be efficient in terms of resources. There are many practices, however, in which the practice manager is not allowed to manage but the partners also decline to take responsibility, alternatively there are practices in which the partners would like to delegate responsibility to a practice manager and for whatever reason the practice manager is not able to respond as they would like. Unfortunately, there are still a number of practices in the latter two groups:

The four partners in the Village Medical Centre realized that they needed someone to organize their practice. The senior secretary, Mrs Jones, was keen to develop her skills. She was encouraged to undertake the course at the local centre, which she completed successfully. Although there was some difficulty accepting her promotion by other staff she soon settled into her role and successfully carried out the partners' policies. After a while problems started to arise, tasks which should have been completed were found incomplete, the partners realized that they were needing to provide more supervision than they felt should have been necessary. It became clear to them that as the practice had developed, Mrs Jones' job had expanded beyond her capabilities. After discussion, the partners agreed that as the practice was entering fundholding there was a need to employ a fund manager with skills to complement those of Mrs Jones and that the new fund manager should take overall managerial responsibility, allowing Mrs Jones to concentrate on administration. Together the partners and Mrs Jones agreed a job description for both posts.

Exercise 15.4   To assess a practice's attitude to practice management

1. What are the current limits of your practice manager's responsibility?

2. Are they included in all partnership meetings, even the delicate ones in relation to income and workload?
   Are they profit sharing?

3. Are they able to hire staff?
   Are they able to fire staff?
   Are they responsible for staff appraisal?

4. Does the practice manager have any restrictions on budget, if so, what are they? Are they the same as the partners?
   Is the practice manager included in all meetings relating to finance?

5. If a new system were needed in your practice, relating almost entirely to administration, would the task be left entirely to the practice manager or would they work closely with one of the partners?

6. Some of the answers to the questions may be influenced by the skills of the present incumbent. If so, what would be the attitude if you were seeking to replace your current manager?

Discussion: It is not uncommon for practices to make internal promotions, it seems less risky to promote a loyal member of staff to a position of practice manager. However, training will be needed if that individual is not to get out of their depth. Sometimes the promotion only works in the short-term and alternative solutions need to be sought. Had this practice not been fundholding their options might have included one of the partners taking responsibility for some aspects of practice management or the use of other resources, such as the practice accountant.

You may like to complete Exercise 15.4 to assess your partnership's attitudes to practice management.

PRACTICE STRATEGY AND BUSINESS PLANNING

One important aspect of practice organization is a clear purpose for the practice —a strategic plan. This plan may or may not help at an operational level for day-to-day activity. It is usually helpful to develop a business plan which brings together strategy and tactics, allowing the overall direction to be maintained but setting clear goals for the short-term with associated likely costs.

All practices are encouraged to develop a business plan, some are more skilled than others in completing the task. Development of a practice strategic plan has been covered earlier in the book. Without clear goals it is difficult to plan practice activity, and the result is likely to be a practice which responds to

Table 15.1 Suggested headings for development of a business plan

Main Heading	Sub-heading
1. Aims and objectives of the practice	
2. Patient services	Current activity Future plans Possible changes in list size Planned introduction/removal of services
3. Partnership structure	Current partnership Possible changes Outside commitments
4. Staffing structure	Current structure Anticipated changes Training needs
5. Building	Possible modifications Upgrading/decorating
6. Equipment	Medical Office Planned upgrading/replacement
7. Review of clinical care	Planned audit and development of protocols Review of secondary care Response to outside pressures, e.g., Health of the Nation
8. Finance	Possible changes Possible ways of increasing income
9. Outside commitments	Clinical sessions Nursing homes

crises rather than one which plans for the future. Business plans vary, they need not be elaborate but they do need to be specific and they do need to include costings where it is appropriate.

Practices will vary in who takes responsibility for a business plan; ultimately one person will need to take overall responsibility, and that person could easily be the practice manager. Time will need to be set aside to develop a plan, and it is likely to take more than one meeting. Individuals should be able to work on aspects of the plan, either alone or in small groups. It is useful to be aware of some general headings when developing a business plan. Table 15.1 shows one way of tackling a business plan. Each section should have a clear plan of activity, an estimated budget, the name of the lead individual and a likely completion data. Table 15.2 shows one way of setting out a business plan. Setting a business plan out in this way allows a practice to consider the overall budgetary implications, and facilitates monitoring activity. If one individual is leading in a number

Table 15.2 A possible layout for a business plan

Area of activity	Objectives	Anticipated budget	Lead person	Completion date
Medical records	Replace torn folders and ensure accurate address and telephone number	10 additional staff hours/week for 6 weeks Total: £300	Senior receptionist	December 1996
Practice computer	Learn how to search for information on the prevention screen	Training day for practice manager and computer manager Total: £500	Computer manager	May 1996
Staff common room	Replace chairs	Replace 5 chairs at £100 each Total: £500	Practice manager	May 1996
Improve care of patients with epilepsy	Update on new drugs Printing of shared care record Postage for clinic appointments Repeat audit	Training course: £100 £600 £25	Dr Jones	December 1996

of areas this may not be realistic, and adjustments may need to be made.

SUMMARY

A well organized practice depends on a number of important factors: strategy, leadership, relationships, rewards, and structure. There are also a number of useful mechanisms which help to keep things running smoothly. A business plan helps to ensure that the strategic vision is implemented; and, although practices may run adequately without a practice manager, an enthusiastic, effective manager co-ordinating and leading practice organization is a great asset.

REFERENCE

1. Stott, N. *The nature of general medical practice*. London: Royal College of General Practitioners, 1995.

16 Staffing

INTRODUCTION

At one time, businesses had workers. Later they became personnel, and these same workers are now named human resources. It is easy to be cynical about such changes in nomenclature. However, the underlying reason for such names is the way in which we value those people who do work for us. 'Our staff are our greatest asset' is a noble part of any company's vision and values statement! The development of human resources as a sub-speciality of business management has also led to a language peculiar to that breed. As with other disciplines (including our own profession), jargon is partly there to exclude others (creating a mystique) and partly to facilitate communication between fellow professionals (a short cut to understanding). However, there is nothing to be frightened of in other people's jargon; the application of a little understanding and a lot of common sense makes it all come clear.

You might hear someone talking about 'skill mix'. In our language, are you employing the right grade of staff to do the jobs you, as a team, need to have done? Or are you employing a practice manager who relieves on reception work? Are you employing a Grade H Nurse to run your phlebotomy service? Another buzz phrase is 'vacancy factor'. This is used to refer to the savings that a practice makes when a post lies vacant. In other words, if a member of staff resigned and you were able to continue to run reception without appointing another for six months, you would save six months of a receptionist's salary.

These sort of phases, apart from irritating us, do two things. They alert us to the ways in which other businesses have made a science out of staff management and how businesses have used that science to achieve more appropriate staffing levels; and they tell us that staffing is an expense on the business and that expense can be controlled (one should properly say, be managed). Of course, managing staff is about much more than money. A brief résumé of staffing issues must include:

- appointment procedures
- job descriptions
- pay and conditions
- contracts
- disciplinary matters
- redundancy
- health and safety
- appraisal
- training.

So you can see that this is not an area to be trifled with. Curiously, general practitioners made a business out of trifling with many or all of these staffing issues for many years. Some still openly flout health and safety regulations (and occasionally get caught). Most of us would admit to a fragmented approach to training and appraisal. We need, therefore, an ordered approach.

FUNDING

Family Health Service Authorities (shortly to be just Health Authorities) provide practices with a budget for staff costs. Although each FHSA sets its budget differently, the value of that budget tends to be between £9 and £10 per patient on the list. However, the FHSA only hands this over when the practice has paid it out, and it does this in a rather odd way. The FHSA is not prepared to pay out more than 70 per cent of what the practice staff costs. Also, the FHSA will only reimburse certain types of staff. The Statement of Fees and Allowances (Red Book) details these types, although the FHSAs do have some discretion these days.

Let us take the example of a practice with a list of 4000 patients which employs:

1 practice manager @ £16 000 p.a.	=	£16 000
1 nurse part time @ £8000 p.a.	=	£8000
1 secretary part time @ £4000 p.a.	=	£4000
3 receptionists part time @ £4000 p.a.	=	£12 000
	TOTAL =	£40 000

The FHSA will reimburse 70 per cent of £40 000 which is £28 000. However, this practice can be reimbursed up to a maximum of £40 000; in order to receive this full allocation, this practice would need to spend £58 000 on staff. Of this, £40 000 would be reimbursed, and the practice would bear the residue as a practice expense. Assuming this practice is profitable, and paying tax at 40 per cent on some of its income, the cost to the practice of employing its current staff is £7200; but if it employs its full quota its costs only rise to £10 800. In other words, the practice can employ an extra £18 000 of staff at an extra cost to themselves (after taking tax into account) of £3600. Exercise 16.1 will help you to clarify these issues in your practice.

SKILL MIX

The chances are that the practice team is like it is because it evolved that way. Evolution is a good way to proceed. Start with too few staff and increase as necessary, when defects become apparent or when the workload rises. But how do you known when that staff complement is not ideal? During good times—no staff sick, none on holiday, none away on training—no defect may be apparent. It is only when a system comes under stress that it fails, for example when a

---

Exercise 16.1   To identify and achieve an optimum staff complement

1. What is your practice wages bill, and what is your staff budget? Are you making full use of your budget?

2. Describe the existing staff complement. Why is it like that?

3. What is the sickness record of your staff?

4. Outline three problems you have spotted that could mean a skill mix problem. Propose a solution.

5. Does each member of your staff have an up-to-date job description?

6. You are about to interview for the post of medical secretary. Who will interview and why, and what will they ask?

---

receptionist breaks a leg during a walking holiday, or when a staff member takes maternity or paternity leave. These are the times to watch for signs that the establishment is not big enough, or not big enough in one area. Of course it may be too big in others! (How many free appointments does your nurse have?) Another sign of a system under stress is, of course, illness. In Exercise 16.1 you could look at your staff's illness record.

If you think there are problems with your skill mix, how do you design a better one? Large companies, and some general practices, use workforce evaluation studies (formerly called time and motion). For most partners, this sledgehammer may be unnecessary; you must, however, identify the area in which you perceive a problem, be it reception, clerical, secretarial, managerial, or clinical. You must then get an idea of the scale of the problem, which will often require an audit. This will indicate the expected size of the remedy. At this stage you might for example have arrived at the following:

Perception of problem: referral letters rarely get out the day they are dictated; sometimes they leave three days later.

Audit: 38 percent of referral letters take more than 24 hours to be typed.

Proposed solution: either release secretary from duties which can be done by a clerk (changing the skill mix) or increase secretarial time.

Try the fourth point in Exercise 16.1 in your practice.

JOB DESCRIPTIONS AND APPOINTMENT PROCEDURES

You have identified a need for a new post or a different post. How will you set about obtaining the right person to fill that post? Here are some questions that you must ask:

1. What is the purpose of this post?
2. What are the duties of this post?
3. What competencies are essential?
4. What qualities must this person have?
5. For how long is the post required?
6. How much am I going to pay for this post?

Much time can be wasted in the selection process by failing to identify the answers to these questions at the start. Nothing is more dispiriting than appointing someone with the wrong skills to a post whose purpose is unclear and this is as true for the employee as for the employer. A job description will provide all the answers to these questions and ensure that applications only come from those who are willing and able to fill the post.

Additionally, a properly constructed job description aids both employee and employer when it comes to answering questions in an appraisal such as: 'Which parts of your post do you feel you do well, and which not so well?' Furthermore, in the inevitable disputes over demarcation between staff, the job description allows the employer to correct under and over working in respective jobs. Question 5 in Exercise 16.1 asks you to check that your staff have current job descriptions.

Now that you are happy with your job description it remains to advertise the post and to appoint a candidate. How will you advertise? This depends on the nature and status of the post. For example, in advertising for a receptionist, one might place an advert in the job centre and a local paper. For a fundholding manager, you might place an advert in a national newspaper with specialist pages, or even use a 'head-hunting agency' to seek the right person.

Applications will be made, and you will have to decide which candidates to invite for an interview. Short-listing can be a random process, but can also be made more rigorous if you use the job description as your bench mark. If previous reception experience was a necessity do not short-list those who have none, however attractive their application may be. (If you were willing to accept those without such experience why did you put it in the job description?) How many will you want to interview, and who will attend the interview? Who will ask questions and which questions will they ask? Do not be afraid to test skills. If you need a typist, ensure that the candidates can type by a typing test! (some people tell lies).

In a restricted labour market, you may be prepared to compromise for a candidate who is not ideal. This approach is fraught with difficulty. If you really need a post to be filled it is still better to re-advertise if the first trawl is unsatisfactory. When you have agreed on the successful candidate, you will offer a post. It is usual to offer a post verbally and when a verbal agreement is reached, to make a written offer which should be accepted in writing. Ensure that your letter is clear, that it confirms the offer of appointment, the start date, the job title and description, and the initial period of appointment. You will also wish to draw their attention to arrangements for appraisal and confirm that a contract of employment will be drawn up.

Don't forget induction procedures. Throwing staff in at the deep end is demoralizing and leads to mistakes. Someone in the practice should have devised an induction and training programme and this should be adhered to. Only when a staff member is happy to commence full duties should he or she be let loose.

PAY AND CONDITIONS

Salary is, in many ways, the easiest part of pay and conditions. Most practices still use Whitley Council pay scales because the FHSA views these as appropriate and will not usually reimburse a practice for an excess payment. Some practices, however, especially those who have difficulties recruiting staff, seek to reward staff in other ways. Although uncommon, this practice has merits. What every practice wants is committed, loyal staff who do not leave lightly. Constantly advertising and appointing new staff is demoralizing. Some practices with a high turnover of staff, symptomatic as it is of a staffing malaise, might consider reward mechanisms. You might consider some of these in Exercise 16.2.

APPRAISAL AND TRAINING

Appraisal is central to staff development. Too often, appraisal is poorly structured and seen as a tool by the employer to address problems with a staff

---

Exercise 16.2   To consider staff development

1. Consider the following and comment on how they might be achieved and what would be the cost and benefit.

   a. workplace crèche facilities

   b. pensions

   c. performance related pay.

   Try to think of other loyalty incentives for staff.

2. How does the appraisal process work in your practice? How did it get like that?

3. What training has your staff received in the previous year? How was this decided? How did the practice benefit and at what cost?

4. Who is responsible for the disciplinary process amongst your staff? How has this been tested?

member. Although that would certainly be part of an appraisal process, it is not all of it. Proper appraisal is planned and is a cooperative process by which the employee can be helped to fulfil his or her potential. Such an approach is valuable to the employer as well as the employee because it enables the employer to match the needs of the practice to the wants of the individual. The process is:

1. Timetable of staff appraisal.

2. Preparation by both appraiser and appraisee, preferably on a written proforma.

3. First the employee and then the employer get a chance to say what is going well and what not so well. Finally, after discussion around these matters, there is a negotiation of an action plan which encompasses training needs matched to the aspirations of the individual and the practice.

Appraisal has nothing to do with the disciplinary process, nor to do with contract negotiations. If it is seen in that light it will fail, since employees have nothing to gain from it (Exercise 16.2). Training needs identified through appraisal should be met. These are the needs of the practice for a new skill in a member of staff and are matched to individual members of staff, so that the most appropriate individual gets the training. The FHSA training budget is often arbitrary and inadequate. Practices should set aside training money in their budgets for the year and go through a process of ensuring that the allocation of training is fair and sensible. For instance, a practice may decide that its priority for training is for the practice manager to learn health and safety law. This will be time consuming and expensive so little training money is available in that year for others. In the following years, though, the needs of others must be considered.

CONTRACTS AND DISCIPLINE

Employees are entitled to a contract of employment, which is a clear agreement between the employer and the employee about the nature, terms, and conditions of the employment. The vast majority of employees in general practice now have a contract, including registrars. A very full description of a contract is given in the excellent BMA book, Employing Staff, which also discusses in depth disciplinary action. In many senses, the disciplinary content of the contract is the most important since few employers or employees study the document until a conflict arises.

Nobody likes disciplining staff (see question 4 in Exercise 16.2). In the small work environment of most practices, news of a disciplinary action spreads fast and morale will be lowered. Everyone tends, at least superficially, to be friendly, and sides are taken which corrupt the way in which work is carried out in the practice. Although discipline has to be exerted, the need for formal action can often be obviated by a good appraisal system which picks up problems early and remedies them. It is, though, essential that the practice knows what it should do in the event of a problem and follows the contractual procedure to the letter. Failure to do so will result in an appeal against unfair dismissal and may lose the practice money and reputation.

HEALTH AND SAFETY

The employer has a duty to protect the employee, and the employee has a responsibility to look after himself and others. This simple statement is enshrined in an enormously complicated law which gives great power to the Health and Safety Executive. The duty of the employer includes a requirement to produce a health and safety Policy Statement (if there are five or more employees—which means most of us) and to inform the staff about health and safety. The law is widely flouted, yet the penalties for failing to observe it range from heavy fines to closure of the workplace. In general practice, because of the hazardous nature of some of the procedures that staff carry out, certain other conditions apply. This regulation is called Control of Substances Hazardous to Health. In addition, employers must maintain an accident book and conduct inspections of their premises to identify risks. You might like to attempt Exercise 16.3.

CONCLUSIONS

As a partner in a practice, you cannot regard staffing as someone else's problem. You work with the team and their morale and happiness will fundamentally influence your contentment at work. You have legal and moral responsibilities which you should be aware of, and attend to. A little time spent on staffing, in ensuring that all have contracts and that appraisal is in place, can often save many hours of heart breaking effort later.

Exercise 16.3 To consider health and safety

1. Where is your practice's Health and Safety Policy Statement? Have you, as the employer, read it?

2. What is COSHH and how does it affect your practice?

3. What is the last entry in your accident book? What action was taken to ensure there was not a repetition?

4. Who conducted the last inspection of your premises and when? What action have you taken?

---

17 Practice accounts

INTRODUCTION

Practices are businesses and as such have to satisfy their 'shareholders' that the business is conducting itself in a secure and sensible way. In the case of general practice, those shareholders are the partners who own the capital of the business, so it is doubly important that the practice demonstrates to itself that it is financially sound. However, there are other interested parties:

1. The Inland Revenue, who want you to pay tax and must know how much the practice has earned;

2. The Department of Health, who want to know how much of the taxpayers' money is being spend and how.

You may feel no inclination to let either party know anything. However, in the case of the Inland Revenue you have no choice; and in the case of the Department of Health it is in the interests of other GPs that they know how much it costs to run the business of general practice so that allowances which reimburse average running costs are set correctly each year. Practice accounts are, however, much more than just a fulfilment of a moral or legal obligation. A proper accounting procedure is the most powerful management tool a business can have. The production of management information from the accounts enables rational financial decisions to be made. Without proper information from the accounts, management decisions are liable to be arbitrary or based on guesses and this will hurt your pocket.

THE PRACTICE ACCOUNTANT

An accountant is much more than a number cruncher. A good accountant will present the accounts in a manner that assists their interpretation; will negotiate on the practice's behalf with the Inland Revenue; will advise on loans and overdrafts; and will offer advice on all major changes in the practice. Although not a management consultant in the sense of offering general management advice, a good accountant becomes an indispensable part of a practice management team.

It is essential, therefore, that your accountant is knowledgeable and trustworthy. An experienced accountant will work for a number of general practices and will have a deep understanding of the special circumstances of the general practice contract and payment systems. Such an accountant will be pro-active, anticipating the effects of changes on the practice, rather than responding to cries for help. This ideal accountant also commands the respect of all partners equally. While one partner may be responsible for the accounts and will therefore get to know the accountant better, it is essential that the accountant's advice is seen to be impartial. It is undesirable, therefore, that one partner should develop a social relationship with the accountant. The accountant's judgement may not be affected, but the confidence of the other partners in the probity and impartiality of recommendations may be reduced.

While the accounts partner and the practice manager will be in regular contact with the accountant and his colleagues, the partnership will wish to discuss the accounts with the accountant regularly. Usually there is a main annual meeting when the draft accounts for the previous year have been first prepared with other meetings arranged when major changes with financial implications are contemplated.

Every partner will need to decide whether to use the practice accountant or a personal accountant to deal with personal financial issues. A personal accountant can act as a second sounding board on practice matters and can offer confidential advice on personal matters. However, it is cheaper to retain the practice accountant for personal matters and there is the issue of shared liability. Since partners are liable for each others' personal debts, sharing an accountant is one safeguard that a partner is not developing a personal situation which could compromise other members of the practice. The loss of confidentiality is, therefore, a reasonable price to pay for the reassurance.

THE CONTENTS OF THE ACCOUNTS

The practice's accounts tell you:

1. at the most basic level—your income and level of expenditure;

2. at an intermediate level—your liability to taxation, and the profitability of your practice;

3. at best—how your money is being spent, where it is coming from, and how the first might be decreased and the latter increased.

This third level is the one to which we all aspire; at their most sophisticated, accounts can help the young principal to understand the business side of the practice and to make sensible recommendations to the other partners. That is why the partner who understands the finances—traditionally the 'senior partner'—has been perceived to wield extra power in the practice.

The only requirement for keeping accounts is diligence in record keeping. No financial transaction should occur without being recorded. Traditionally, these records were kept in a cash book by a method known as doubly entry bookkeeping, in which each entry is recorded twice; once in a totals column and once in a column that specifies the type of expenditure or income incurred. The reason for this double recording is that it enables a total of all income and expenditure to be quickly calculated while also enabling the totals to be broken into their component parts so that reasons for changes can be deduced. This quite simple concept is the basis for the provision of financial management information. Any modern practice will, by now, have abandoned the cash book for the spreadsheet. This is a computer programme designed to allow a single entry to generate whatever totals and analyses might be required to increase understanding. Although the underlying principles are the same as the cash book, the increased accuracy of calculations and the presentational capacity offer a significant benefit. A spreadsheet account can be transferred onto the accountant's computer, avoiding the re-entering of data and reducing some accountancy charges. For this reason it is important to ensure that your spreadsheet is compatible with theirs, and that the layout of your entries meets the accountant's requirements.

EXPENDITURE

Appendix A shows a set of theoretical practice accounts for one quarter. You might like to consider which items represent the greatest expenditure for the practice. This information is gleaned from the '1/4 total' column. This sort of information is useful on its own, and trends from month to month can be quickly seen. The system improves even more, however, when we add some more information. In Appendix A there is a column labelled 'Budget' which contains a quarter of the practice's best guess for expenditure in the year, followed by two columns which show how the real expenditure compares to the projection. To decide the estimated expenditure, the practice undertook a budget setting exercise based on the previous year's accounts in which some areas of high expenditure were to be reined in to increase profitability. Looking at Appendix A, consider which items have exceeded their budgets and which have made savings at this stage of the year.

Bookkeeping is not quite as simple as it is made to appear here, because there are other needs as well. The accounts book has to be made to balance with the bank statement; this checking process ensures that the accounts represent exactly the money coming in and out of the practice and that no receipts or payments have been missed. This monthly checking process is called reconciliation and is every manager's nightmare.

INCOME

The principal source of a practice's income is the payment that comes from the health commission (which was formerly the Family Health Services Authority). This payment is divided into various categories; the main ones are:

- capitation
- allowances
- items of service
- reimbursements (of rent, staff costs).

Each of these has further subdivisions, and in the case of items of service, there are a large number of subdivisions. Some practices create a ledger in which they record not only the total health commission payment, but break it down into its components. Other practices enter the full details into their spreadsheet. In Appendix B, an analysis of an item of service spreadsheet is shown. As in the case of the cash book, it is useful to know what the expected total is for each item; this information can be established from the health commission (for local averages) and Medeconomics (for national averages). Thus any practice can compare its performance to that of others. This is shown as a 'variance per cent'. You might like to look carefully at Appendix B and consider how this theoretical practice compares to the national average. This management information is vital to the financial health of the practice and will inform its decisions about money and about clinical practice

PARTNERS' DRAWINGS

In simple terms, the partners could, at the end of each month, subtract the month's expenditure from the income and divide the 'spoils' or profit between themselves. This is common and sensible but only if the practice has a clear idea, from information provided by the accounts, about the state of the bank account—that is the cash flow situation. Supposing a practice appears at the end of a month to have a surplus of income over expenditure of £4000, it might choose to simply divide that amount among the partners. But if in the next month there is a substantial bill due, say for income tax, the partnership's bank balance might become very overdrawn. So deciding a reasonable level of partner's drawings will depend on the practice's anticipated cash flow; and a practice can improve its cash flow just as other businesses do:

1. by not paying creditors (people to whom you owe money) until you really have to

2. by pursuing debtors (people who owe you money) for early payment

3. by balancing the costs of personal overdrafts to individual partners against the cost of a practice overdraft with its tax benefits (a practice overdraft is a business expense).

There are, of course, other factors which complicate the situation. Not all partners get the same profit share. On coming into a new practice it is likely you will receive a smaller share for a period of time and this will be specified in the partnership agreement. Part time partners receive lower shares in proportion to their contribution to the practice workload. The calculation of profit share from the residual profit has therefore to be modified by a calculation in percentages.

If a partnership continued to simply divide up each monthly or quarterly profit in shares for the partners, there will be no money left in the practice for development. In other words, the only source of investment income for a practice is the profit. Practices should always underdraw where possible so that a capital reserve is left for contingencies, such as new equipment or repairs. This money still belongs to the partners according to the share each takes of profits and is represented in the final accounts by the term capital account. The alternative is that all capital expenses are met from loan accounts or overdrafts which can lead to overall negative capital accounts for the partners. This is no problem in itself but can cost the practice dearly in bank charges and means that there is no asset value for a departing partner.

Because we work in a partnership, the practice is liable for the collective income tax of the partners and employees. This means that the Inland Revenue calculates the tax due on the 'profit' of the business and the accountant works out what share of income tax each partner pays. However, all the partners are jointly responsible for the tax due; if one fails to pay, the other must do so for him. For this reason, it is sensible for a practice to hold a tax reserve by regular transfer from the practice account, rather than share out all the available income and leave income tax payment to the individual—there are many recorded occasions of partners leaving without paying a tax bill that then falls on the other partners. The monthly partnership tax saving should be large enough to pay all anticipated tax bills in the year ahead, with any fortuitous over-saving divided between the partners or carried forward to decrease the next year's savings.

One further detail concerning the payment of income tax is the 'tax year' on which the business works. A practice can, on the advice of their accountant and with the agreement of the Inland Revenue, choose a date from which its tax year begins. Since the assessment of income tax is done soon after April 5th and is based on the last complete set of accounts, a practice that is becoming more profitable every year will delay payment of income tax by having a tax year from July 1st to June 30th. However, this is due to change over the next three years and all businesses will move to a current year's earning principle. At the end of the tax year, the accountant will come and remove all cash books, receipts, invoices and everything your manager has prepared in relation to the tax year just finished. He collates and checks that information and presents it to the partnership in the form of end of year accounts.

END OF YEAR ACCOUNTS

The end of year accounts are to general practitioners what medical records are to the accountant, that is they are in another language. But you can learn this language and use it to inform your decisions about the practice. In Appendix C, there is a set of illustrative accounts for a two doctor practice. The accounts show two sets of figures: one set for the year just ended and another alongside for the year before that. This enables the practice to compare profitability with the previous year. The accounts consist of a number of sections and each is subdivided.

1. Practice income: (Part C of Appendix C) this summarizes the information provided from the practice, and illustrates its change over the previous year.

2. Practice expenditure: (Part A of Appendix C) this summarizes the information provided by the practice. The accountant has added an element for depreciation in expenditure to account for the loss of value of the fittings and fixtures of the practice. This reduces theoretical profitability and eases the tax burden.

3. Profit and loss account: (Part A of Appendix C) this gives the difference between income and expenditure, with the exception that the money taken by the partners as income is not an 'expenditure' in the sense used here. The balance sheet shows that the practice still has some money in the bank at the end of the year, and was owed some money and the accounts show this on the credit side. On the debit side the practice still owes some money.

The drawings by the practitioners are less than the profit made when all this is taken into account and so the partners have lived within their means and left some money behind for the practice, which adds to their capital accounts (Part D of Appendix C). In looking at the year end accounts in Appendix C, you might wish to reflect on the financial viability of the practice. If the bank demanded the repayment of the loan, would the practice be able to do so? Are the partners drawing too much, too little, or about right?

CONCLUSIONS

This chapter has illustrated the main features of a practice's accounts. Since you are likely to own part of your practice in the near future, it is important that you understand all this yourself rather than have it explained to you. Conflict often arises in general practice between partners when decisions are taken about profit levels, buying in, and partnership shares. It is in your interests to take an active part in those decisions. Mature a relationship with the practice accountant and, if different, your own accountant; ask about financial aspects that you do not understand; and do not agree to substantial changes in the practice unless the financial implications are clear to you. Partners should appreciate a colleague who ensures that the practice makes sound financial judgements.

Appendix A A quarterly analysis of expenditure

	July	August	September	1/4 Total	Budget	Variance	Variance %
Bank interest charges			412.00	412.00	358.50	53.50	14.92
Cleaning, laundry	20.00	63.50	19.00	102.50	88.00	14.50	16.48
Computer expenses				0.00	155.00	−155.00	−100.00
Courses				0.00	159.75	−159.75	−100.00
Depreciation				0.00		0.00	
Drugs/consumables	220.32	110.90	194.62	525.84	571.25	−45.41	−7.95
Heat, light			292.06	292.06	351.75	−59.69	−16.97
Insurance				0.00	110.75	−110.75	−100.00
Levies	6.58	6.58	6.58	19.74	19.75	−0.01	−0.05
Loan interest			2100.00	2100.00	2200.25	−100.25	−4.56
Locum fees		1625.00	410.00	2035.00	3828.75	−1793.75	−46.85
Lease of equipment	30.60	32.72	30.60	93.92	91.75	2.17	2.37
Postage/printing/stationery	220.34	208.62	180.30	609.26	433.25	176.01	40.63
Professional subscriptions	563.00			563.00	541.75	21.25	3.92
Rates on surgery/waste	63.00	43.00	120.32	226.32	478.00	−251.68	−52.65
Repairs/renewals				0.00	111.25	−111.25	−100.00
Staff uniforms				0.00	178.25	−178.25	−100.00
Sundries/accountancy	3420.00	43.20	25.00	3488.20	961.75	2526.45	262.69
Telephone/pager			624.32	624.32	448.25	176.07	39.28
Textbooks/journals	24.20	16.20	16.20	56.60	154.25	−97.65	−63.31
Wages/salaries	3300.00	3280.00	3394.00	9974.00	10 549.75	−575.75	−5.46
TOTALS	7868.04	5429.72	7825.00	21 122.76	34 377.48	−13 254.72	−38.56

Appendix B Comparison of items of service income to national averages

Items of service	National average per patient	Expected total	Practice total	Variance %
Child health surveillance	41.90	1063.84	1088.00	2.27
Contraceptive service	91.00	2310.49	2037.00	− 11.84
Emergency treatment	3.90	99.02	8.00	− 91.92
Health promotion	149.40	3793.27	1125.00	− 70.34
Maternity	142.80	3625.69	3073.00	− 15.24
Minor surgery	46.10	1170.48	—	− 100.00
New registrations	38.30	972.44	2711.00	178.78
Night visits	118.90	3018.87	3051.00	1.06
Temporary residents	34.40	873.42	797.00	− 8.75
Vaccs, Imms—adults	56.70	1439.61	1915.00	33.02
TOTALS		18 367.13	15 805.00	− 13.95

Appendix C Example of year end accounts

A. Overall profit/loss

	This year £	£	Last year £	£
INCOME				
Income from General Medical Services etc.		146 361		122 155
Building society interest		294		383
		146 655		122 538
EXPENDITURE				
Bank interest, charges	1434		953	
Cleaning, laundry	352		2506	
Computer expenses	622		786	
Courses	639		1623	
Depreciation	2744		4095	
Drugs and consumables	2285		3019	
Heat, light	1407		1016	
Insurance	433		441	
Levies	79		81	
Loan interest	8801		8733	
Locum fees	15 315		2967	
Lease of equipment	367		367	
Motor expenses	2028		3159	
Postage, printing, stationery	1733		4247	
Professional subscriptions	2167		2795	
Rates—surgery, waste disposal	1912		1919	
Repairs, renewals	445		1275	
Staff uniforms	713		435	
Sundries including accountancy fee	3847		4655	

Expenditure (*continued*)

Telephone, pager	1793		2866	
Textbooks, journals, periodicals	617		444	
Use of house	624		715	
Wages, salaries	42 199	92 566	43 241	92 338

NET PROFIT FOR THE YEAR	54 089	30 200

B. Balance sheet

	This year		Last year	
	£	£	£	£
FIXED ASSETS				
Valuation of assets		109 598		81 434
Surgery loans		(118 985)		(90 028)
		(9387)		(8594)
CURRENT ASSETS				
Debtors, pre-payments	5348		2785	
Cash at bank	4274		5522	
Cash at building society	1563		7909	
Cash in hand	55		17	
	11 240		16 233	
CURRENT LIABILITIES				
Creditors, accrued expenses	5905		5414	
Hire purchase account	—		1375	
	5905		6789	
NET CURRENT ASSETS		5335		9444
NET (LIABILITIES) \ ASSETS		£(4052)		£850
REPRESENTED BY:				
Partners' capital accounts		£(4052)		£850

C. Income

	This year	Last year
	£	£
INCOME		
Basic practice allowance	6444	7740
Standard capitation fees	41 368	48 996
Seniority	385	—
	48 197	56 736
Item of service fees, target payments	18 267	13 886
Postgraduate education allowance	4067	5002
Ancillary staff reimbursement	26 911	25 598
Rates reimbursement	1694	1473
Insurance medicals/private fees	5031	3722
Drugs/appliances reimbursement	2865	1750
Training reimbursement	297	459

Income (*continued*)

Training grant	—	3220
Computer reimbursement—maintenance	1078	499
Cost rent	5280	1320
Notional rent	2800	3900
Medical record grant	—	4500
Medical audit expense reimbursement	214	90
Locum reimbursement	3525	—
Hospital salaries	26 135	—
TOTAL GROSS INCOME	£146 361	£122 155

D. Partner's Capital Accounts

	Total	Dr A	Dr B
PARTNERS' CAPITAL ACCOUNTS			
Balances b/f	850	(825)	1675
Capital introduced	5725	2222	3503
Net profit for the year	54 089	27 045	27 044
	60 664	28 442	32 222
DEDUCT: Drawings	(64 716)	(36 976)	(27 740)
Balance	£(4052)	£(8534)	£4482
Profit shares		50%	50%
PARTNERS' DRAWINGS			
Monthly drawings	40 046	20 023	20 023
Sundry drawings	2900	1714	1186
Superannuation	4395	2955	1440
Income tax/class 4 NIC	10 075	5088	4987
Tax/NI on outside appointments	7300	7196	104
	£64 716	£36 976	£27 740
CAPITAL INTRODUCED			
Practice expenses paid personally	4047	2222	1825
HP re: payments (car) paid	1678	—	1678
Personally			
	£5725	£2222	£3503

18 Premises

INTRODUCTION

The pendulum has swung to and fro on the issue of premises for general practitioners over the years since the inception of the NHS. Before 1946, GPs owned premises, often in their homes, and financed such investment through payments from patients. After 1946, things changed slowly, but in the 1960s, with the advent of reimbursement of rents, there was a boom in Health Centres owned by District Health Authorities (now part of commissioning authorities) which rented accommodation to practices. That situation still persists in many areas (particularly cities). However, most GPs now own their premises again and by doing so build up a property investment at very little cost to themselves, by virtue of the reimbursement they obtain. There are three ways in which a GP can hold premises from which to practice. Each has its merits and it is up to the individual to decide the path along which to travel. A practice can rent from a private landlord (who might be one of the partners); rent from a health authority; or own their premises. These three options will be examined in turn.

RENTING PRIVATE PREMISES

The practice enters into an agreement with a landlord for suitable accommodation. It might be a genuine commercial landlord or it might be a partner in the practice. The health commission (previously FHSA) sends a District Valuer (a public servant) to assess the market rent—a reasonable rent for the property—and agrees to reimburse the practice for this on a monthly basis. If there is a disagreement between the landlord and the District Valuer, the commissioning authority will usually arbitrate and it is usual for the practice to end up with a no-cost situation.

The advantages of such an arrangement are that the practice ties up no capital and is not responsible for the upkeep of the fabric of the building. Further, it can be easier to attract a new partner where there is no capital investment involved in joining the practice. The disadvantages are that the practice is not building up a capital asset heavily subsidised by the health service (see below). Rented accommodation is usually multi-purpose—for example a converted house—which the landlord could rent to a non-medical business should you leave; therefore the premises are often not ideal for primary care. Lastly, the practice does not control the development of the premises. If new staff are to be accommodated, the landlord must be persuaded to extend the building.

RENTING HEALTH CENTRES

In this option, which was very popular in the 1970s and early 1980s, the health authority builds premises which are designed for primary care, and the practice rents them. Since the health authority reimburses the practice its rent, there is a paper transaction for the rent between two parts of the health commission, with the practice left only to fund the costs of heating, light, and maintenance. Although the practice is not involved in paying and claiming back rent, the process is explicit since it needs to appear in the practice accounts on both sides as income and expenditure. The advantages of a health centre are that the premises are purpose-build, sometimes to a high standard, sometimes not, with no rent to pay. Against this option, the practice is not building up capital, it can be very difficult to persuade a health authority to invest in extensions, and health authority interest in funding these schemes has markedly declined.

BUYING PRIVATE ACCOMMODATION

Practices can own their premises as a partnership. This may be an old surgery which has been extended over the years or it may be a converted house or office. More and more common are purpose built premises on a new site. A practice that builds its own premises with the agreement of the health authority will have much of the cost reimbursed (see below). It, therefore, builds up a capital asset with little investment by the practice and each partner can sell their share on retirement. This reality has to be tempered with the fact that increasingly the costs of new premises outstrip the capacity of the funding schemes to reimburse practices, and many practices contribute significant sums (but much less than the full cost) towards their premises. A practice which owns its own premises is, however, master in its own house and can apply to the health commission for access to funding schemes to allow it to extend. Many practices prize this autonomy. On the debit side, premises are a responsibility which need looking after, and they can be subject to a negative equity trap—the loans taken out to build can exceed the market value.

When a partner leaves, prospective replacement partners might be put off by the need to invest. This is an important issue for this book, since readers may confront this exact position. Just as a young doctor is planning to take out a large mortgage for a house, it seems hard to be expected to invest heavily in practice premises. However, the incoming partner acquires both the capital asset of the outgoing partner and the eligibility for cost or notional rent (see below). A bank will finance the premises purchase while the health commission reimburses costs of the interest payments (not the capital repayments); under most circumstances the actually cost, in monthly cash terms, for the incoming partner is minimal. This does, however, make a quick change of mind more difficult and may involve some complex arrangements (facilitated by the accountant) if the practice was built quite a while ago; each doctor must decide if gaining a substantial capital asset cheaply is worthwhile.

FUNDING PREMISES

Practices that are being charged a fair rent, as agreed by the District Valuer, and who are receiving reimbursement for that rent, do not need funding for their premises. For those who own their own premises, there are three financial packages to understand.

Notional rent

The simplest scheme to understand is notional rent. If a practice owns their premises they are paying no rent. But, theoretically, they could be renting their premises to another business and working from other premises which they rent —with the rent being reimbursed to them. In the interests of equality, the Department of Health agreed to reimburse a practice what it would have been charged if the premises were not owned by the practice. So the District Valuer decided on a fair rent and the health authority reimburses that sum to the practice.

In reality, most practices in this position have outstanding loans for buying or extending the premises, but as far as the health service is concerned, that is their business. They can borrow commercially at favourable rates (practices are regarded as safe bets) and it is clearly in their interests to keep the repayments less than the notional rent. As time goes by, the notional rent increases with market rents (it is reappraised every three years) and the practice borrowings do not keep pace (if major extensions are undertaken, improvement grants come to the rescue—see below). The practice keeps the difference as divisible income.

Cost rent

If a practice decides to move out of its accommodation and to purpose build new premises, the repayments on the interest on the capital cost will definitely, at first, exceed the market rent as decided by the District Valuer. This meant that the new build option used to be very expensive for practices, and in practical terms was not viable. Hence the introduction of the cost rent scheme.

If a practice wishes to enter this scheme it must first approach the health authority for outline permission. Funds for cost rent schemes are limited and practices must justify their eligibility in comparison to others. If permission to proceed is given, the practice finds a site and obtains planning permission. It employs an architect to design the premises and the architect then invites tenders from builders for the job. The architect costs the project completely, including all professional fees involved. The commissioning authority and the practice agree on the price and the practice then obtains finance from a lender, usually the General Practice Finance Corporation or a bank. The building work goes ahead and at the end of the project the total costs are assessed.

An illustration of a cost rent scheme

In this example, a 20-year-loan of £120 000 would cost the practice per year:

Interest set by the bank at 7 per cent over 20 years	=	£7200
Straight capital repayments over 20 years	=	£6000
TOTAL COST	=	£13 200
Less cost rent reimbursement	=	£9600
DEFICIT	=	£3600

The health authority then uses Department of Health set rates to assess the level of reimbursement to the practice. For example, supposing the total cost of the project was £120 000 and the practice has obtained a loan from the bank for the whole amount on a variable rate loan (which varies with the current bank rate); and supposing that the variable cost rent rate is 8 per cent (determined by the General Practice Finance Corporation rate at the time). The health authority will reimburse the practice £9600 per year, which represents the interest on the loan. The practice must pay the capital itself, but in reality, since the variable rate is often set more generously than the rates at which practices can obtain loans, there is often only a small cost to the practice. Above, this example is worked further, in which a rate of 7 per cent has been negotiated but a reimbursement rate of 8 per cent applies (a not unreasonable supposition).

In this case the cost of each partner in a two partner practice of acquiring a £60 000 asset is £1800 per year, and this cost is reduced by using endowment or savings plans to repay the capital. However, every three years the District Valuer will be asked to re-value the premises and determine a fair rent. As soon as that rent exceed the reimbursement from cost rent (and the interval varies according to the buoyancy of the office premises market) the practice switches to notional rent. Not only will this be more than the cost rent, but it will increase every third year in line with the District Valuer's assessment. There are complications that can make the scheme look more complex, but no less attractive:

1. The variable rate of cost rent is reviewed annually in the light of prevailing interest rates.

2. The health authority can offer a fixed rate of cost rent repayment so that practices can take advantage of lenders willing to offer short-term fixed rates. Fixed rates offer a practice longer term stability so that regular outgoings can be calculated and this improves a practice's cash flow.

3. Health commissions sometimes use a combination of rent and cost rent to calculate a practice's reimbursement for premises. This flexibility can help a practice.

4. The change to notional rent is irreversible and requires an accountant's advice.

5. The health authority uses nationally set bands to determine the maximum cost of a building that it will reimburse. For example, London practices would obtain higher limits than rural ones because of the relative prices of land. Larger practices have higher limits than smaller ones. The Red Book (Statement of Fees and Allowances) contains all these limits, which are revised annually.

The cost rent scheme takes a lot of a practice's time and attention. The building and occupation of new premises are not a scheme to be undertaken lightly. At all stages, from initial consideration to final occupation, the health authority has to be consulted and their agreement sought.

IMPROVEMENT GRANTS

The Red Book sets standards for practice accommodation. In some cases, practices wish to remain in their accommodation as it is, but would want to improve facilities for the practice and patients. In such cases the health authority will make grants of up to 66 per cent of the cost of such improvements. These cash grants are one-off payments designed to encourage GPs to improve services without too large a cash burden.

Schemes for which the FHSA is allowed to make grants include:

- Bringing into use new rooms not currently used by the practice
- Improvements to lighting and heating
- Double glazing
- Provision of car or pram park
- Improvement of toilet or washing facilities
- Improved disabled access
- Security systems

but the rules in the Red Book are tight on the exact improvement and the reason for it.

As with cost rent schemes, an approach to the health authority in the first instance will ensure that they have available the funds within their budget (there is a cash limit on the overall sum available for improvement grants) and will agree to your proposed scheme. Proper plans must be presented and the practice has to guarantee to continue to use the premises (or forfeit the grant if they do not). If the practice does not move within three years of receiving the improvement grant, this sum is not repaid, and there are no further financial implications involved in accepting it. Of course, the practice must fund the remainder of the improvement with a loan; however, the new improved premises are assessed for the notional rent by the District Valuer on his next visit, and the improvement may increase the reimbursement through that route.

STANDARDS

A practice is unlikely to want to move to new premises, however attractive the reimbursements may be, if there is no problem with the existing practice. But how do you know if your premises are adequate? The Red Book contains a section entitled *Premises—minimum standards*, which refers in general terms to the requirements the FHSA has before it will offer reimbursement to a practice under any of the premises schemes. These general requirements are specified more clearly in respect of new premises under the cost rent scheme in the section on cost rent in the Red Book. These more specific requirements can be used as a guide to good practice in terms of the quality of premises.

CONCLUSIONS

Our working environment is very important—for ourselves who will spend many hours in the surgery, for our primary care team who have to tolerate its inadequacies, and for the patients who frequent it. Premises effect the morale of the practice, the range of services it can offer, and its quality of care. In this chapter, the ways to finance premises have been explored. Although not necessarily straightforward, they do offer the opportunity to work in good surroundings at little cost to the practitioners.

19 Technology

INTRODUCTION

Technology is 'the practice of the applied sciences that have practical value or industrial use' according to *Chambers' twentieth century dictionary*. In this section we shall take this to mean the way in which we use science to help us run our general practice business. General practice, indeed the whole business of health care in hospitals and outside, has been slow to introduce new technology. Many of the systems in everyday use in general practice have been present for very many years without change. Some practices still use card index systems to excellent effect to compile, for example, morbidity indexes. Most practices still use paper accounting procedures, and most practices issue monthly pay slips to their staff that have been worked out on a calculator and transferred onto paper. Some practices still write repeat prescriptions by hand.

The use of older technology to assist in the running of a practice is not necessarily a bad thing. If a system works, why change it? However, as a new principal, you will need to be able to make an assessment of the procedures in your practice to judge their effectiveness and efficiency (Exercise 19.1). You need to ask first if the current, low technology methods of working are adequate and then, if you are not content, to decide how technology can best be applied. However, even if the answer is that you and the practice are quite happy with the way the practice runs, you still need to ask if technology could help things to be done quicker, better, or cheaper. There are certain areas in which most general practitioners will use technology to some extent. You may want to add others, but these core areas must be considered:

- patient care
- financial management
- word processing
- graphic design
- communication.

Exercise 19.1   To consider the role of technology in your practice

1. Where is your practice on the technology ladder? Rate this from 1–10 (1 no technology, 10 everything).

2. Is this where it needs to be?

3. How did it get where it is?

4. What drives or impedes progress?

PATIENT CARE

In Chapter 14 the role of the computer for tne electronic patient record was explored. However, technology extends into patient care far beyond the clinical record and its databases. A practice might decide that its care of diabetic patients is not ideal; many diabetics might have proteinuria on stick testing and are in danger of sliding into renal failure. The practice decides to start screening for microalbumiuria and needs to invest in kits to do so. Or, a practice decides that it wants to screen for glaucoma and must invest in tonometers and training.

It is worth reviewing the equipment we use in day to day patient care. A simple way to do this is to get each partner to make a note each time he or she wished to do a procedure but didn't have the equipment to hand. Over a three month period a recurring pattern may develop; a common theme about the absence or poor quality of the equipment present. Equally, it is useful to talk to others in the practice who may not have such a say in the way things work. In particular talk to the nurse ('I've been moaning for years about that ear syringe') and to the secretaries and clerks. They too have a voice. Increasingly, practices are considering the need to have a defibrillator, nebulizers, tonometers, near-patient biochemical and bacteriological testing, a sigmoidoscope, cautery, or syringe drivers. Your practice may have many other items of patient care technology.

Patient care is the focus of all our activity. Most technology is used to directly enhance patient care while other technology based systems are there to support us in delivering patient care. We are beholden to our patients to ensure that we use the most appropriate and effective system for their benefit.

FINANCIAL MANAGEMENT

The purpose of financial systems in a practice is explained in Chapter 17. However, the mechanism by which financial information is provided needs consideration. In essence, a practice has to decide what its need is for financial information. In many small, non-fundholding practices employing few staff that need may be very small. In such practices, it may be sufficient for a single handed partner to keep simple paper accounts. In larger and more complicated practices, there is a greater need for more detailed knowledge of outgoings and income, because more partners need to share that information and there is a greater capacity for mismanagement.

Traditionally, a business records its financial dealings in a form known as double entry bookkeeping. Although this was, historically, always done by hand in an accounts book, there has been a trend towards computerized accounts which mirror the double entry method but do the adding up for you, and are able to present the information in a readily comprehensible form. The program which computers use to do this is called a spreadsheet.

The inexorable development of computer financial accounting systems can be confusing. At its simplest, a financial package consists of a table, just as one would draw up on a piece of paper. Each row and each column can be given a title (for example wages, electricity). The package allows the user to record in each square, or cell, a value just as the user would do in the accounts book. The spreadsheet keeps a tally of changes and adjusts the value at the end of each column and row. This simple explanation does no justice to current systems on offer which can also produce reports such as 'trend of electricity bills last eight quarters', or 'trend of maternity service income last four quarters', far quicker than could a manual system. A computer accounts system that calculates salary, tax, National Insurance, prints pay slips, P45 and P60 can be obtained for less than £100. If your practice manager still spends three hours per month (the minimum for a manual system) doing these calculations by hand, and you already have a personal computer, you need a wages package.

WORD PROCESSING

There is nothing mysterious about word processing, although the suppliers of the software would have us believe so. We all have to write letters, reports, and so on and the word processor is just a way of doing this. The chief benefits are:

- no need to retype a whole document each time corrections are made
- no need to print out until perfect
- better and more flexible presentation of documents
- the ability to preserve the skeleton of a frequently used document (template)
- the ability to save the document on disc rather than keep a file paper copy
- the ability to send the same letter to a group of people at different addresses without having to retype it each time (mail merge).

The use of word processing in general practice is very variable. Some practices do not use typewriters at all, and have minimal paper filing systems—all referral letters are filed in the patient's computerized record. Others use typewriters for referrals but use a word processor for reports. Others do not use a word processer at all. Some GP computing systems have excellent word processing systems included. Others are frankly awful, so that a typewriter is better and easier to use. The computer market is awash with systems that cost from £5 for a shareware system to £500 for combined design and write systems. In between are excellent word processors that cost only £100 and have so many features that you will never use them all.

GRAPHIC DESIGN

This section is concerned with the way in which we present ourselves to our customers. Good presentation is good for business; a business that appears half hearted in its presentation is seen as half hearted in its conduct of that business. Well presented documents with appropriate embellishment go a long way to selling a business and this is where technology can help.

All GP's must now produce a practice leaflet. This leaflet is not only a statutory requirement; it is also seen increasingly as a marketing tool. Although a practice can, and most of us still do, order printed stationery and leaflets from a printer, the technology exists to do it yourself. A word processor with a design package and a good printer will produce stationery, leaflets and advertisements to the same or better quality than a professional printer. Additionally, you have the flexibility to change your presentation as often as you wish, since you only produce it as you need it. Computer programmes that produce complex documents with graphics are called 'desk top publishers'. They require training and time before a member of staff can be fluent in their use, but they justify the effort.

COMMUNICATION

We receive and we pass on information; this communication is time consuming and expensive. It is, nevertheless, essential. Errors in communication are not uncommon and cost even more time and money. Of course, our communication systems need to be near perfect when we are dealing with patients, but we need to apply the same standards to communications in general if our working lives are to be efficient.

Telephones and faxes

The first area to consider is the humble telephone. Telephone bills absorb a high proportion of a practice's expenses. The market in telecommunications has meant that prices have come down but practices can save more money by using Mercury for long distance calls. Avoiding out-going calls at peak times and using faxes (see below) when passing on complex messages can help.

A mobile telephone can transform your life. Equally it can make your life very miserable. The calls are still very expensive, and the networks still not 100 per cent reliable. It can, however, allow you to respond to an emergency message immediately, without the need to find a public telephone. And many general practitioners extol its benefits for calling patients requesting an emergency visit to assess the call; to call patients when you cannot find their house; and for dealing with those small domestic problems that add to the stress of a weekend on call. If you want to be more available to your staff and your patients, you can afford it, and you have a back-up system, then it is worth using a mobile telephone. Obtain competitive quotes (don't forget that the purchase price is the smallest component; recurrent costs are the worst bit) and develop some rules about how the phone will be used and by whom.

It is cheaper to fax a letter than to post it. It gets there quicker and you know it's got there. That is not to say that you will save money by having a fax; the capital cost will take a while to recover. There are other caveats—private and confidential letters that you would not want a secretary to see can't be faxed, and bulky documents are better posted. Also, there is no fax equivalent to recorded delivery.

Most practices find that the real advantage of having a fax machine is as a receiver of messages. The pathology laboratory will fax a result which is needed quickly without you hanging on the phone or a secretary trying to understand the values which the lab dictates to them. An insurance company will fax forms which the patient forgot to bring (and you will fax back the result so a decision gets made without delay). The FHSA will accept a faxed claim form at the eleventh hour for any maternity claims you forgot to send. Once you have one, you can't live without it. Practices usually start by attaching the fax to an existing line, but the constant bother of turning the line over to the fax machine will mean they quickly order a separate line with a separate fax number.

Electronic data transfer

This is the big issue for the near future. Already, personal computers compose fax messages on screen and then send them to a distant fax machine without a paper version even existing. If the distant fax machine is, in fact, another computer with a modem—a device that connects the computer to a telephone line—then the 'fax' is in fact an electronic message. Soon fax machines will be superseded by electronic messaging. Such messages can be set up by one computer dialling another using the conventional telephone numbers or it can be through networks as electronic mail, or e-mail. For this, each computer linked to the Internet has an 'address' that identifies its location. A distant computer dispatches a message attached to that address into the network and soon—usually within a few hours at the most, much less when the network is quiet—it arrives at the recipient computer. When you switch on your computer, your local network computer tells you that that you have e-mail and there it is. Long documents can be sent through e-mail as well as short notes.

E-mail is not very confidential and for most medical purposes we will continue to use direct modem links. Within a short time—and this is a reality in many practices already—all communications from hospitals such as pathology reports, discharge summaries, out-patient letters, and death notifications will arrive electronically; and the health authority will conduct its business with the practice, such as registering or removing patients and receiving items of service claims, through an electronic link.

When a user is making regular contact through telephone lines with another site, as would be the case between a main and branch surgery or between a surgery and the local hospital, the speed of conventional telephone lines may become frustrating. In this case the line can be upgraded to ISDN-2 standard which greatly increases its capacity. Communication with a distant computer becomes almost instantaneous.

COSTS AND BENEFITS

Technological advance has both costs and benefits. In particular, recurrent costs are often bigger than capital costs. For every innovation that you consider you need to draw up a realistic list of the following costs:

- hardware; the costs of the machinery you buy
- software; the costs of the programs you buy
- recurrent costs; upkeep and materials (for example fax paper)
- training
- health and safety; new technology means new rules
- time; convincing people is hard work! but after that you will need to invest time in ensuring the technology is being used most effectively.

Against those costs you need to enumerate the expected benefits. Technology has a reputation for replacing people but this is seldom the case in general practice—the advantage lies in a job being done better and any released staff time is usually quickly absorbed elsewhere. However, you will want to consider these possible benefits:

- better patient care
- easier clinical audit, health needs assessment, and business planning
- more accurate information
- more timely information
- more effective communication
- a better image.

CONCLUSIONS

Exciting new technology of today is the routine technology of tomorrow. Throughout a working life in general practice new developments will challenge that practice's capacity to afford and use it effectively. A wise practice follows the innovators and carefully appraises the technology to ensure that it will complement its care, not imperil it. History suggests, however, that appropriate technology can help us to enhance the quality of the patient care we deliver—and that should be the prime yardstick when assessing a new technology.

20 Going forward

INTRODUCTION

The contents of this book have been arranged in a deliberate order. First, we looked at how we have arrived at where we are and where that is; then we looked at the major problems a young principal faces and studied some solutions; and, lastly, we have looked at real skills and knowledge that help a young principal to make an effective contribution to their practice. In this short, last chapter we will draw together a number of threads that have permeated this book.

CLINICAL CARE

General practitioners are, first and foremost, clinicians. They are, in fact, the general physicians of the health service today, carrying the pivotal role in patient care. It is true that they do not carry this task alone; they have increasingly numerous and sophisticated primary care teams and they have many referral agencies, not least the hospital. However, it is the general practitioner who has the guardianship of the patient's medical record, who orchestrates care, and who advocates for the patient within the health and social services.

As management in primary care becomes more competent, the general practitioner of tomorrow will spend more time on patient care which will be concentrated on those problems that require the high level skills of a doctor. Nurses and therapists will take over more and more patient care for which they are trained, with doctors using their hard won skills more effectively. And increasingly, patients will look to the practice to offer many medical services that even now are regarded as the province of secondary care.

So, the general practitioner of tomorrow will have to acquire, develop, and retain high level skills. This requires a long-term commitment to continuing medical education, evidence based medicine, and quality assurance. In the latter task, the role of clinical audit will undoubtedly grow, with patients, colleagues, and health service managers seeking to be reassured that we all continue to deliver high quality care.

THE GENERAL PRACTITIONER AS MANAGER

Management cannot be avoided, although it can be controlled and minimized. A modern general practitioner is at the centre of a primary care led health service, commissioning care for individual patients and for the practice population. The practice needs to be managed as a business with financial, staffing, and administrative issues to be addressed. A general practitioner has to make choices and live with the results—often for years. Some management choices have profound clinical implications: is a physiotherapist a better use of resources than several hip replacements? Other choices affect the quality of a patient's experience of care in the practice: should the practice invest in new premises? Increasingly, general practitioners are supported by highly professional practice managers and need only concern themselves with the general principles and monitoring their implementation. However, it is difficult to make good decisions on principle without understanding how the practice works. Every general practitioner needs to be a manager.

DEVELOPING AS A PERSON

In order to deliver high quality care, the family doctor needs to develop himself or herself. This means developing a greater understanding of people and patients, and reaching forward to new levels of communication. It also encapsulates the need to seek and find interests which expand the intellectual horizons so that daily consulting is enriched. Many achieve this through vocational training and teaching undergraduates, others gain it through clinical assistantships or external appointments. It is not necessary for these activities to be medical and many general practitioners achieve an excellence in fields unrelated to medicine.

Patients expect that their doctor will be a balanced human being, with wide experience of life and with a variety of interests. A young principal may find the task of integrating into a new practice consuming enough for many years, but will in time wish to develop as a person beyond the strict limits of the task of being a general practitioner. This book has offered some guidance on the choices.

Every practitioner will, however, wish to grow and not diminish as the years go by. This will require supporting relationships within and outside the practice and an ability to cope with the very real stress of modern day general practice. The ability to develop in ways that are not self-destructive and which enable the doctor to help others to develop likewise is to be cherished.

CONTRIBUTING TO THE DEVELOPMENT OF THE DISCIPLINE

All the members of a discipline, and we belong to the academic community of general practice, benefit from the vibrancy and development of that discipline. There are many levels at which this can be achieved. A general practitioner can enhance the reputation of general practice through the quality of care delivered in the practice. This is the most important contribution any of us can make. As a discipline we have other needs. We need evidence on which to base our clinical and managerial decisions, and that evidence is best derived from research. We need committed teachers, both undergraduate and postgraduate, of high quality in order to enhance the skills base in primary care. And we need intellectual leaders, be they medical politicians, local committee chairmen, or those who offer new insights into our work. Few of this years entrants into general practice will become leaders in any of these three fields. But if they contribute to the communal effort by taking the odd student in the practice, collaborating in a research project, or putting forward views in a logical and constructive manner, the discipline will be enriched.

ENJOYING IT

If all these elements can be put in place—high quality clinical care and management, personal and professional development, and contribution to general practice as a whole—then a young general practitioner will stand an excellent chance of eventually looking back on a successful and happy career. We all have a responsibility towards our colleagues, helping them to reach fulfilment in their working lives but also offering support, compassion and understanding—as we would to any patient—if they fail, sometimes fleetingly, to get job satisfaction. We, the authors, hope that you have seen how much general practice has to offer, and what skills will enable you to maximize your pleasure from a remarkable vocation.

Appendix 1: Departments of General Practice

Professor J Bain, University Dept of General Practice, University of Dundee, Westgate Health Centre, Charleston Drive, Dundee. **Tel: 01382 644425**

Dr C J Bulpitt, Clinical Tutor, General Practice Education Activities, Royal Postgraduate Medical School, Hammersmith Hospital, Du Cane Road, London, W12 0HS. **Tel: 0181 743 2030**

Dr P D Campion, Department of Primary Care, University of Liverpool, Whelan Building, PO Box 147, Liverpool, L60 3BX. **Tel: 0151 794 5597/8**

Dr G Fowler, University of Oxford, Dept of Public Health & Primary Care, Gibson Buildings, Radcliffe Infirmary, Woodstock Road, Oxford, OX2 6HE. **Tel: 01865 511293**

Professor R C Fraser, Department of General Practice, University of Leicester, Leicester General Hospital, Gwendolen Road, Leicester, LE5 4PW. **Tel: 0116 2584871 (direct)**

Professor G Freeman, Department of Public Health & Primary Care, 4th Floor, Chelsea & Westminster Hospital, 369 Fulham Road, London, SW10 9WH

Professor P Grob, Department of General Practice & Health Care Research, Robens Institute, 29 Frederick Sanger Road, Surrey Research Park, Guildford, Surrey, GU2 5YD. **Tel: 01483 509203**

Professor A Haines, Department of Primary Health Care, University College & Middlesex School of Medicine, Highgate Wing, Whittington Hospital, Highgate Hill, London, N19 5HT. **Tel: 0171 272 3070 ext 4607**

Professor D R Hannay, Professor of General Practice, Department of General Practice, University of Sheffield, Medical School, Beech Hill Road, Sheffield, S10 2RX. **Tel: 0114 7715414**

Professor C M Harris, Professor of General Practice, Division of General Practice, School of Medicine, University of Leeds, Leeds. **Tel: 0113 2334179**

Professor R Higgs, Professor of General Practice & Primary Care, King's College Hospital Medical School, Bessemer Road, London, SE5 9PJ. **Tel: 0171 346 3016**

Professor S R Hilton, Department of General Practice and Primary Care, St George's Hospital Medical School, Cranmer Terrace, London, SW17 0RE. **Tel: 0181 672 9944**

Professor R Hobbs, Professor of General Practice, Department of General Practice Medical School, University of Birmingham, Edgbaston, Birmingham, B15 2TJ. **Tel: 0121 414 6764**

Professor J G R Howie, Department of General Practice, University of Edinburgh, Levinson House, 20 West Richmond Street, Edinburgh, EH8 9DX. **Tel: 0131 650 2807**

Professor B Jarman, Department of General Practice, St Mary's Hospital Medical School, Norfolk Place, London, W2 1PG. **Tel: 0171 723 7169**

Professor R Jones, Department of General Practice, UMDS, Guy's & St Thomas' Medical & Dental Schools, 80 Kennington Road, London, SE11 6SP. **Tel: 0171 735 8881**

Professor A L Kinmonth, Department of Primary Medical Care, Faculty of Medicine, University of Southampton, Aldermoor Health Centre, Aldermoor Close, Southampton, SO1 6ST. **Tel: 01703 783111**

Professor D Mant, Department of Primary Medical Care, Aldermoor Health Centre, Aldermoor Close, Southampton, SL1 6ST. **Tel: 01703 783111**

Professor B McAvoy, Department of Primary Health Care, University of Newcastle upon Tyne, The Medical School, Framlington Place, Newcastle upon Tyne, NE2 4HH. **Tel: 0191 222 6000 ext 8761**

Professor B W McGuiness, Centre for Primary Health Care, School of Postgraduate Medicine, University of Keele, Thornburrow Drive, Hartshill, Stoke-on-Trent, ST4 7QB. **Tel: 01782 716047**

Professor T S Murray, Department of General Practice, University of Glasgow, Woodside Health Centre, Barr Street, Glasgow, G20 7LR. **Tel: 0141 332 8118**

Professor T O'Dowd, Department of Community Health, Trinity College, 199 Pearse Street, Dublin, Ireland. **Tel: 00 3531608 2293/1087**

Dr N Oswald, Director of Studies in General Practice, University of Cambridge, Clinical School Offices, Addenbrooke's Hospital, Hills Road, Cambridge, CB2 2QQ. **Tel: 01223 336723**

Professor D J Pereira Gray, Department of General Practice, University of Exeter, Exeter Postgraduate Medical Centre, Barrack Road, Exeter, EX2 5DW. **Tel: 01392 431159**

Professor M Pringle, Department of General Practice, University of Nottingham, Queen's Medical Centre, Clifton Boulevard, Nottingham, NG7 2UH. **Tel: 0115 924 9924 ext 01394**

Professor P Reilly, Department of General Practice, Queen's University, Dunluce Health Centre, 1 Dunluce Avenue, Belfast, BT9 7HR. **Tel: 01232 240884 ext 252**

Professor L D Ritchie, Department of General Practice, University of Aberdeen, Foresterhill Health Centre, Westburn Road, Aberdeen, AB9 2AY. **Tel: 01224 681818 ext 53971**

Professor M O Roland, Department of General Practice, University of Manchester, Rusholme Health Centre, Walmer Street, Manchester, M14 5NP. **Tel: 0161 256 3015**

Professor W Shannon, Royal College of Surgeons of Ireland, Department of General Practice, Mercer's Health Centre, Stephen St Lower, Dublin 2. **Tel: 00 0178354**

Professor D Sharp, Professor of Primary Care, General Practice Unit, Department of Social Medicine, University of Bristol, Canynge Hall, Whiteladies Road, Bristol, BS8 2PR. **Tel: 0117 928 7319**

Professor L Southgate, The Academic Department of General Practice & Primary Care, St Barts & London Hospital Medical Colleges, New Science Block, Charterhouse Square, London, EC1M 6BQ. **Tel: 0171 982 6100**

Professor N C H Stott, Department of General Practice, University of Wales College of Medicine, Health Centre, Maelfa, Llanederyn, Cardiff, CF3 7PN. **Tel: 01222 541133**

Professor P Wallace, Professor of Primary Care & Population Sciences, Royal Free Hospital School of Medicine, Rowland Hill, London, NW3 2PF. **Tel: 0171 794 0500 ext 4760**

Dr J F Wilmot, Senior Lecturer in General Practice, School of Postgraduate Medical Education, University of Warwick, Coventry, CV4 7AL. **Tel: 01203 523913 (direct)**

Appendix 2: Regional Advisers in General Practice

Dr G B Taylor, Regional PG Inst for Med & Dent, 10–12 Framlington Place, The University, Newcastle Upon Tyne, NE2 4AB. Tel: 0191 232 8511 ext 7029

Dr J Bahrami, Postgraduate Dean's Office, 1st Floor, West Wing, Yorkshire Health Buildings, Park Parade, Harrogate, HG1 5AH. Tel: 01423 567117

Dr E A Birkby, Dept of Postgraduate Medicine, Faculty of Medicine & Dentistry, Univ of Sheffield, Medical School, Beech Hill Road, Sheffield, S10 2RX. Tel: 0114 2712526

Dr R Hedley, Postgraduate Office, Medical School, Queen's Medical Centre, Nottingham, NG7 2UH. Tel: 01602 709377 ext 44473/41377

Dr D Sowden, GP Postgraduate Education Dept, Leicester General Hospital, Gwendolen Road, Leicester, LE5 4PW. Tel: 0116 2588119

Dr R M Berrington, The GP Office, NHS Executive, 2nd Floor, Central Block, Fulbourn Hospital, Cambridge, CB1 5EF. Tel: 01223 218777

Dr P Pietroni (Acting Reg Adviser), British Postgraduate Medical School, Commonwealth Bldg, Hammersmith Hosp, Du Cane Road, London, W12 0HS. Tel: 0181 743 0367

Dr N R Jackson, British Postgraduate Federation, Central Office, University of London, 33 Millman Street, London, WC1N 3EJ. Tel: 0171 831 9618/9622

Dr L A Ruben, BPMF Office, UDMS, Guy's Campus, St Thomas Street, London, SE1 9RT. Tel: 0171 955 4434

Dr R G Hornung, Stirling House, Stirling Road, Guildford, Surrey, GU2 5XH. Tel: 01483 579492

Dr D Percy, Wessex Regional Health Authority, Highcroft, Romsey Road, Winchester, Hants, SO22 5DH. Tel: 01962 863511

Dr J C Hasler, The Medical School Offices, John Radcliffe Hospital, Headington, Oxford, OX3 9DU. Tel: 01865 221520

Professor D J Pereira Gray, The Regional Advisers Office, Dept of GP, Postgrad Med School, Barrack Road, Exeter, OX2 5DW. Tel: 01392 403023

Dr R C W Hughes, Dept of Postgrad Medical Education, Univ of Bristol, Academic Centre, Frenchay Hosp, Frenchay Park Road, Bristol, BS16 1LE. Tel: 0117 975 7050

Dr A Lewis, Department of General Practice, Exeter Postgraduate Medical School, Barrack Road, Exeter, EX2 5DW. Tel: 01392 403023

Dr D Wall, West Midlands RHA, GP Unit, 142 Hagley Road, Edgbaston, Birmingham, B16 9PA. Tel: 0121 456 1444 ext 1700

Dr A G Mathie, Postgraduate General Practice Office, Hamilton House, 24 Pall Mall, Liverpool, L3 6SL. Tel: 0151 236 2637

Dr J Hayden, Department of Postgraduate Medical & Dental Education, Gateway House, Piccadilly South, Manchester, M60 7LP. Tel: 0161 237 2104

Dr Simon Smail, Dept of PG Med & Dent Education, University of Wales, College of Med, Heath Park, Cardiff, CF4 4XN. Tel: 01222 743059

Dr Agnes McKnight, Northern Ireland Council for Postgraduate Medical Education, 5 Annadale Avenue, Belfast, BT7 3JH. Tel: 01232 491731/4

Dr H I McNamara, Postgraduate Medical Centre, Raigmore Hospital, Inverness, IV2 3UJ. Tel: 01463 234151 ext 5201

Dr W Reith, Aberdeen Postgraduate Centre, Foresterhill Medical School, Aberdeen, AB9 2ZD. Tel: 01224 681818 ext 53976

Dr R F Scott, PG Division, Level 8, Ninewells Hospital & Med School, Dundee, DD1 9SY. Tel: 01382 60111 ext 3140

Dr W M Patterson, Lister Postgraduate Institute, 11 Hill Square, Edinburgh, EH8 9DR. Tel: 0131 650 8085

Professor T S Murray, West of Scotland Committee for Postgraduate Medical Education, The University, Glasgow, G12 8QQ. Tel: 0141 339 8855 ext 5276/4738

Brigadier M Conroy, MOD, Army Medical Directorate, Room 21.50A, Building 21, Keogh Barracks, Ash Vale, Aldershot, Hants, GU12 5RR. Tel: 01252 340345

Wing Commander Webb, Institute of Community & Occupational Medicine, RAF Halton, Aylesbury, Bucks, HP22 5PG. Tel: 01296 623535 ext 7652

Air Cdre Keith Prior, Institute of Community & Occupational Medicine, RAF Halton, Aylesbury, Bucks, HP22 5PG

Surgeon Captain R D Curr, RN Sick Quarters, HMS Drake, Plymouth, Devon, PL2 2BG

USEFUL ADDRESSES

Royal College of General Practitioners, 14 Princes Gate, Hyde Park, London, SW7 1PU

British Medical Association, Tavistock House, Tavistock Square, London, WC1H 9JP

Index

Italic numbers denote references to tables, figures and/or exercises.